A Million Things To Ask

Easy

"Loved it... For anyone into the basics of the science of the brain and fiery neurons filled with questions on how this super organ works and controls the human body, this is one fascinating read... Complex neuroscience mechanisms are explained with daily life examples... It is almost like being in an exciting classroom with an amazing teacher who brings the subject home... This book is a thrilling ride and literally food for thought."

- Aneesha Shewani, Reedsy Discovery

"Made me laugh out loud... I am the first to admit that I do not have a scientific bent of mind, and normally, I shy away from anything that smacks of science. But Dr. Tranter explains things in a way even the most non-science-oriented ones (like me) can understand... He has some comments that made me literally laugh out loud. The "X-files of neuroscience" segment was even more intriguing than the question/answer segment."

- Long and Short Reviews

"Fascinating... I like the choice of topics. They are not too quirky, and revolve around everyday things- dreams, brain freeze, addiction, bilingualism, for example... It's friendly and simple enough that even someone like me can easily follow up the narration. The last part, where we're going, is fascinating."

- Viviana-MacKade Reviews

"A surprisingly funny and engaging read... The book is both down-to-earth and full of humor as he explains in simple terms how our brains work. A Million Things To Ask A Neuroscientist is a perfect book for the budding scientist in your life to the curious reader... Everyone will find this book interesting and delightfully brimming with strange facts about our brains."

- Hurn Publications

"Give this book a look...Within its pages you will be entertained and informed. Readers learn about the common and the uncommon in an approachable manner... So, if you want to learn if it's possible to increase your IQ, how to effectively multi-task, what causes depression, or have other beguiling questions answered, give this book a look."

- Travel The Ages

A Million Things To Ask A Neuroscientist

A Million Things To Ask A Neuroscientist

The Brain Made Easy

Mike Tranter PhD

Book design by Madeeha Shaikh (DezignManiac)

Edited by Selena Class

ISBN 978-0-578-86169-2 (paperback)

www.aNeuroRevolution.com

6 7 8 9 10

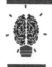

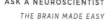
TABLE OF CONTENTS

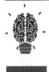

TABLE OF CONTENTS

3. THE FUTURE OF NEUROSCIENCE

4. DOWN THE SCIENCE RABBIT HOLE

5. WOMEN IN STEM

PREFACE

OK, you got me. There isn't actually a million questions in this book, but there is the *possibility* to ask a million questions. That is what I love so much about science – you can always ask something new. Even if you revisit the same old problems, it can be you who discovers something new. That spark, excitement and curiosity, to find the answer for no reason other than because it is there to be discovered, is what makes a great scientist. Simply by picking up this book and challenging yourself to learn about the brain, you have shown that same curiosity. You don't need to be a nerdy scientist in a laboratory like me to find that spark of joy, that excitement for the strange and novel, and the curiosity for answers. That is a fundamental human trait and one that will be given free rein in this book.

I spend most of my life in a laboratory researching how the brain works. I find a tremendous sense of joy in what I do, but the opportunity to talk about the brain's inner life with people and why it does the things that it does brings me the greatest joy. This is the first book that I have written, and it has been so much fun to write. Interacting with people from all over the world who are curious about science has filled me with genuine excitement and amazement, which is hopefully demonstrated throughout the following chapters.

When I first decided to write this book, I wanted it to be guided by the ideas that really sparked people's sense of wonder. So, I asked people worldwide to submit their most interesting questions about the brain – questions that they have always wanted to know but never had the opportunity to learn about. I have been surprised and humbled by the amount of support and interest that people have shown. The response surpassed even my highest expectations and allowed me to look at science from a different perspective. To learn what other people find fascinating about the brain, and their interest in neuroscience, would inspire me throughout writing this book.

As I am from England, in the UK, I made my social media name 'The English Scientist', I know, not very original. Staying true to form, I made sure to use the British spelling of words, partly for British pride, but mostly for the amusement of my American friends and colleagues when they read drafts of this book.

It was a challenging process to narrow down the best questions to include. Some are given their own section, while others are included in the text's body, which allowed me to tailor the content to what you asked for. The responses and enthusiasm were so great that I expanded the book with additional chapters designed to give you an inside peek into other areas of neuroscience, to look at it from the eyes of people actually doing the research – a viewpoint that few people outside of the lab really get to see. We will explore how neuroscientists are using our current understanding of the brain to create a new and futuristic world for humanity that could almost be straight out of a science fiction novel. We will lift the lid on the inner workings of the brain and show you what happens when it doesn't work quite the way it should, and also explore how science permeates so many different facets of our life.

The final chapter, written by Jodi Barnard (née Parslow) is dedicated to women who study and work in STEM (science, technology, engineering and mathematics). It was important for me to add this chapter as I have seen first-hand, with friends and colleagues, some of the challenges women face when establishing themselves in a career as a scientist, not only in research but in all fields. I am incredibly proud and lucky to have this bonus chapter written by Jodi - a promising woman in STEM today, as she shares her perspective on how to be an incredible scientist. I hope it encourages and inspires you to keep pushing your limits and to never stop learning.

Thank you again for reading my book and showing your support. Now let's get on with it, because as I always say......

science never sleeps!

Introduction

A Quick Look Inside the Brain

What is our brain? Yes, it is the pink mushy thing inside our head that helps us to communicate, to learn new things, to keep us awake at night worrying about that awkward joke we told a week ago, to... well, do almost everything – but what exactly is it?

The brain is the control centre of everything that our body does, almost all of which is controlled outside of our conscious mind so we don't even have to think about it. We don't consciously control when we are hungry or tired, or when to change our blood pressure or heart rate, and we certainly don't tell ourselves to feel pain when we stub our toe. The brain does all of that, and considerably more every second of the day, even when we sleep.

The Neuron

Without getting too detailed just yet (I don't want to scare you away), let's talk about what our brain is actually made of. You are probably aware that the brain consists of brain cells, called *neurons*. These are the cells that send signals (called *action potentials*) all over the brain and connect with other brain cells in an extraordinarily complex and ever-changing network. An estimated 88 billion neurons exist in your brain, and each one can have thousands or tens of thousands of endings, which form *synapses* when connected to other neurons.

Impressed yet? Well, how about when I tell you that some of these neurons can send action potentials at nearly 300 miles per hour? That's faster than a Formula 1 car! A typical neuron is drawn below and consists of a cell body containing the nucleus (it stores the DNA and dishes out instructions), an axon (the railway the train of signals travels along), dendrites (which are like the smaller railways going to specific places) and the synapse (the mediaeval drawbridge where the railway stops and messages are thrown over the gap). That's it! That's all there is to a brain cell, and now you know about one of the most important cells in the body, you are officially a neuroscientist.

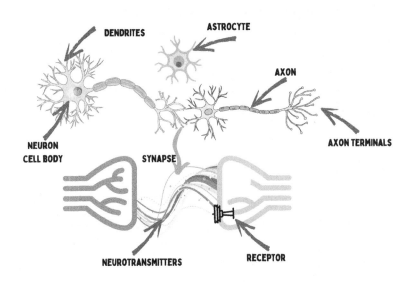

The dendrites of the neuron will form connections with others. These connections, will result in a synapse where the neurotransmitters are released. The axons can also be coated in myelin to make the electrical signals travel more efficiently.

NEUROTRANSMITTERS

At the synapse, *neurotransmitters* are released. These are chemicals that do just as advertised – they 'transmit' a signal between neurons. Because the synapse is essentially just a gap between neurons, they need a way to send messages across, and so neurotransmitters are released. When an action potential travels along one neuron it eventually gets to the end, where the signal causes the release of a neurotransmitter. When the second neuron receives it (it binds to specialised *receptors* that 'catch' the neurotransmitter), the neuron knows to carry on the signal – like a relay runner handing over the baton. These signals, which are nothing more than coded electrical messages, will give our brain instructions. This could be to recall a memory, to laugh at a joke or to fall asleep – anything really.

You may have heard of some neurotransmitters already, such as serotonin, dopamine, noradrenaline (norepinephrine) and glutamate. They basically represent the languages of the brain. Some neurons speak the language of dopamine and some speak serotonin, for example. It is a way for our brain to talk to the areas that it wants, such as the dopamine-speaking parts, rather than let the entire brain hear the message, which would only confuse it.

OTHER BRAIN CELLS

When scientists talk about the brain being made up of neurons, they actually tell a little bit of a lie: it also consists of other types of brain cells such as *glial cells*. The brain has nearly 10 times as many glial cells as it does neurons. The term glial cell is a broad term for a number of specialised cells. For example, microglial cells act like our brain's immune system because our normal immune cells and antibodies, would be far too destructive if let loose in the brain. Glial cells also develop into a specialised cell type called an *astrocyte*. Around 25–50% of our brain is made of astrocytes, which means we have up to five times more of them than neurons. Astrocytes are supportive cells that float along right next to neurons and help out any way they can. They also do many things for themselves, such as creating structure amongst the cells, absorbing and releasing neurotransmitters just like the synapse does, and promoting the formation of a barrier called the *blood-brain barrier*. Other cells include the *ependymal cells*, which create cerebrospinal fluid (CSF) that protects the brain and remove wastes products, and the *oligodendrocytes*, which are a type of cell that coat the axon of a neuron with *myelin* to help it transmit signals better. You don't need to know too much about them for now. We will go over them later, but it gives you a good idea that there is a lot more than just the typical brain cell in that brain of yours.

THE BLOOD–BRAIN BARRIER

If you read about the brain, you will often see people talking about the blood-brain barrier, or BBB. In short, the blood in our body is the transport system for everything. The blood vessels act like the road system we drive on every day. Just like the roads, our blood carries all sorts of traffic, like cars (red blood cells), emergency services (the immune cells), food trucks (food particles, fats, proteins, sugars, etc.) and criminals on the run (bacteria, viruses). The brain is too important to be involved in all of this action, so a barrier is formed between the blood supply for the rest of our body and that specifically for the brain. Oxygen, glucose and red blood cells all pass through easily, but bacteria, immune cells and just about everything else, do not (although there are times when they do cross over and this is bad news for our health). The BBB is one hurdle that we, as scientists, have to cross (literally) when we want to create drugs that target the brain. As great as it is at protecting the brain, it also causes issues with getting medications across.

WHITE AND GREY MATTER

All of the cells mentioned above are broadly grouped into either *white* or *grey matter*. They are named this way because there is a subtle difference in colour between them, with one looking more greyish than the other. White matter is seen within the spinal cord and deeper levels of the brain. It is made from the long axons of the neurons and gets its white colour from a fatty substance that coats them called myelin. The myelin helps to insulate the cell. White matter also contains a lot of astrocytes.

Grey matter is predominantly found in the outer layers of the brain and in the cerebellum. It contains the cell bodies of the neurons, the dendrites, many glial cells and smaller blood vessels called capillaries. The grey matter is the control hub for the neurons and where all of the clever brain power comes from. Although white and grey matter can be defined by the regions of the brain and spinal cord in which we find them, there is also some overlap, meaning that you can get sneaky little cell bodies and glial cells even in white matter.

This is what our brains are made from. Now you know. Keep this in mind when someone tells you that the brain is a muscle – you can tell them how very wrong they are, and explain what the brain really is.

DIFFERENT BRAIN REGIONS

All of these structures and cells that we have just learned about are organised in a very sophisticated way. Our brain loves organising, but with it comes a style of compartmentalising that has taken millions of years to develop. This means that although the brain generally works as a single-unit 'whole brain', there are regions (called *lobes*) that are specialised for specific tasks. The brain is comprised of four major lobes (plus the minor insula and limbic lobes). They each have their own jobs to do before connecting with other regions to share the responsibilities. Although they can be divided into smaller regions (around 180), these four lobes give you a good idea of how your brain is organised.

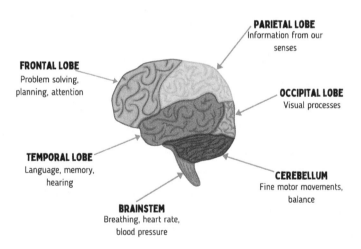

PARIETAL LOBE
Information from our senses

FRONTAL LOBE
Problem solving, planning, attention

OCCIPITAL LOBE
Visual processes

TEMPORAL LOBE
Language, memory, hearing

CEREBELLUM
Fine motor movements, balance

BRAINSTEM
Breathing, heart rate, blood pressure

The typical lobes of the brain. Don't worry about them too much for now, we will talk about them later.

6

Introduction

Throughout this book, you will notice some 'sciencey' words to describe the different areas of the brain. In most cases, they are simplified so you only get the important stuff and don't get bogged down with all the science terms. Sometimes though, there is no way around it – I had to use them. Have no fear though, because if you ever forget what they mean, there is a helpful glossary at the end of this book that you can refer to whenever you need. You can also ignore the word and pretend like it doesn't exist – either way is good.

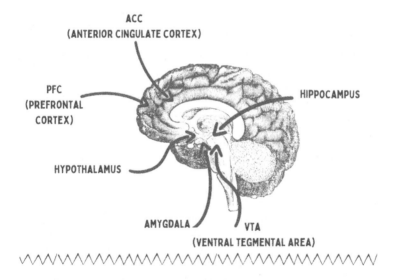

Here is a guide to the general locations of some of the more important areas of the brain that come up throughout the book. Don't worry though. You don't need to know what these words mean if you don't want to. They are here in case you feel like referring back to them at any point, to help visualise where things are happening in the brain.

How it is all connected

Often in neuroscience we talk about one part of the brain or one neurotransmitter at a time. We do this because they have an essential role in something that the brain does, but in reality, they never act alone. The brain is connected to different regions by trillions of connections to create an incredibly complex system that we are not even close to understanding yet. Throughout this book, we will discuss these connections. Simply put, a connection refers to how the neurons talk to each other. They don't just send a message to one neuron and then switch off for the night. They talk to thousands of other neurons, which in turn speak to another few thousand, which creates a network of connections. What neuroscience is starting to tell us is that our brain works the way it does not only because of differences in brain regions but also because of how the brain is connected to other areas. As you will discover in this book, our brain is unique to every individual person in how it connects to other regions. No two brains are quite the same, because however it works, it is unique to you.

At any given moment, there are literally billions of brain cells talking with each other. Considering that visual processing takes up around 65% of all brain activity, just think how many brain cells are working together right now while you are reading this sentence. What a great time to read some more. Let's go!

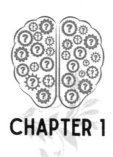

CHAPTER 1

ASK A NEUROSCIENTIST

WHY IS THE BRAIN IN OUR HEAD AND NOT SOMEWHERE ELSE?

It seems reasonably consistent in nature to put the brain in the head (but not always). Why is our brain not somewhere else in our body? In fairness, some do suggest a man's brain is somewhere else, but I don't think the neuroscience backs that up entirely. Wouldn't the brain be safer if it was protected by our ribcage, or out of the way of any danger in our leg or foot? As horrifying as that would look, the answer is relatively straightforward.

First, let's think about the head. The brain relies on sensory inputs – information from our senses about what we see, smell, hear, taste and touch. Vision accounts for nearly 65% of all brain capacity, and so it makes sense to have the eyes as close to the brain as possible. If the brain is placed away from our primary senses, it will cause a small, yet critical, delay in receiving the information. A delay of only a few milliseconds (a thousandth of a second) could historically have meant the difference between life and death. The brain wants all the gossip about what's going on around it, and it likes to be at the centre of everything, so the faster it can be told the information, the better it feels.

But wait, couldn't the senses just form around the brain, wherever it was placed? Throughout the millions of years of evolution from our water-dwelling ancestors to humans, the brain ended up in our head, at the top of our body. If you think about fish, mammals or insects, the head is usually the region where the animal first encounters the world around it as it moves through its environment. It would be a big advantage to have our senses reaching out into the environment around us to interpret the world before proceeding. Getting that information faster would keep us safe from predators and give us an advantage when searching for prey. As humans, our brain, and therefore our senses, perch high above our environment to provide us with the best view of everything around us – and remember, although the brain is a little exposed in this way, it is protected by a quarter-inch of skull, the toughest material the body can produce. So, it should be safe.

WHAT IS THE OLDEST PART OF OUR BRAIN, AND WHAT DOES IT DO?

When we think about how the brain has evolved, it is often explained as a sort of three-brain model. One brain is our reptilian brain, another is our emotional brain, and then there is our superior genius brain that is our neocortex, which I like to call Gary. But how true is all of this, and why do I have a reptile brain sitting next to Gary?

This conceptualisation of the brain comes from a neuroscientist called Paul MacLean, who in 1990 fully detailed his *triune brain theory*.[1] He claimed that the early brain evolved from fish and later reptiles. At this stage, it contained only the basal ganglia, and eventually the brain stem and cerebellum. These parts form the older brain, often referred to as the reptilian brain, which is responsible for the more primitive functions of life – things like thirst and hunger, sexual drive, the impulse to protect our territory, aggression, heart rate, breathing and body temperature.

There are countless books, articles, memes and commentaries about how this reptile brain rules our life and how we need to overcome it to improve our behaviour. They detail how to stop us from acting out with aggression or impulsive behaviour. There is some truth to that, but in general, it is not how the brain works. As we are about to discover, that view is a little outdated. Yes, the reptilian brain would have been the first 'type' of brain to evolve (at least in terms of what we now think of as a brain). These basic functions, such as thirst and hunger, would have kept us alive,

11

just like they do today. But throughout evolution, other parts of the brain have formed around it, as a sort of extension of this reptile brain. This is different from the idea that we have additional, more intelligent brains, simply added on top like building blocks. The brain grew and developed more complex processing power, rather than separate brains added later. We know this because of how well the brain works as a complete structure, with every part of it integrated as one brain.

When we evolved, the first brain extension would have been the midbrain and limbic system,[a] which support emotions, motivation and long-term memory, amongst other things. These two areas would have been important throughout our evolution as we learned to make social connections, and build civilisations and communities, helping us to live with other people and understand the world around us.

As time went on, we developed the neocortex. This is the outer part of our brain, with all the folds (gyri) that you may have seen in pictures of the brain. Those gyri help to shape the brain in a way that increases its surface area, allowing more neurons to be condensed into each area and improving our cognitive processes and connectivity, making us smarter. The neocortex is responsible for a lot, such as our conscious thoughts, planning and reasoning skills which elevate the human brain above those of other animals. This is why it is often said that our neocortex can override our more basic instincts and emotions. Think of it a little like a nagging friend, always thinking they know right (and they usually do) and trying to get you to take a deep breath, relax and think about

[a] The term limbic system itself is fiercely debated in neuroscience because nobody can decide which parts should be included, but for the time being, we will call it the limbic system, and not worry too much about it

things before steaming in with your first reaction. In reality, although that nagging friend has the final word, each region of our brain is well connected to the areas around it – meaning there is no primitive brain giving instructions, only initiating the thought before it is rapidly integrated by the entire brain.

For many years, scientists thought this neocortex distinguished human beings as the 'all-dominant' species because our neocortex is where the really smart areas of our brain go.

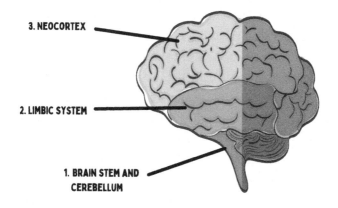

The brain evolved to have more complex integration of different regions.

Neuroscientists once believed that having a large neocortex created our intelligence and was responsible for the humans we are today. Actually, what we see is that other mammals also have a neocortex. Even the size of the brain isn't very big in humans, not when you compare it to that of a large mammal like a whale. However, what distinguishes humans is the ratio of brain size to body weight: humans have a 1:50

ratio, meaning our body weighs 50 times more than our brain (about 1.4kg or 3lbs). That is a remarkable ratio as we have dedicated a lot of our total body weight to the brain. Most mammals have a ratio of around 1:180. So, relative to our size, the brain is about five times bigger than we would expect it to be. With the help of the gyri, it is the organisation of the neocortex which explains why our brain, and especially our neocortex, is so impressive.

To give some context to how far we have come from our water-dwelling ancestors, the neocortex of modern-day humans has been subdivided into approximately 200 different areas. Early mammals with little or no neocortex would have had 20, maybe less, and with very poor organisation.

So, back to the reptilian brain and impulsive behaviours and emotions. Early neuroscience – based on MacLean's view – believed that these older brains acted independently. When you act out in anger, that is the reptilian part of your brain, but when you gaze into the cosmos and wonder about our existence, that is the neocortex working. We now understand that this isn't exactly true. Because our brain evolved to develop more functions, and with it, a bigger size and different shape, all parts of our brain are connected in a way that wasn't really appreciated in the 1960s. The regions within the reptilian brain do initiate those immediate thoughts and impulses, but because the brain works as a whole organ, those feelings serve to trigger a larger, whole-brain effect. Like turning the ignition key to start a car, sure it may start the engine, but the car only drives off because the entire car works together, the driver included (the driver being the neocortex in this analogy).

For example, anger is a very complex emotion. It relies on our memory, future predictions of an outcome, context and physiological stress, amongst other things. It is too simplistic to say 'my reptile brain made me do it'. The early three-brain model is not entirely wrong though, because it is possible to override basic drives such as hunger, threat detection and negative emotions by applying further reasoning and context to the situation. The reptilian brain areas serve the same primitive functions as always, but they are too well-connected to act alone. So, yes, we do have older parts of our brain that help with the basic function of life, but they have also developed into a modern-day brain.

WHAT DOES CANNABIS ACTUALLY DO TO MY BRAIN, AND SHOULD I BE WORRIED?

All drugs are harmful in some way. Not just the ones we take for recreational use, but the ones developed in a laboratory too, like those made by pharmaceutical manufacturers and prescribed by your doctor. Drugs that come from plants, such as cannabis, have a massive amount of chemical components to them and we barely know how many of these work (but that is part of the fun of science – there is always more to figure out).

Cannabis, particularly THC (tetrahydrocannabinol, the primary psychoactive compound in the Cannabis sativa plant), works by binding to receptors throughout the body – the CB_1 and CB_2 receptors. CB_2 receptors are found on immune cells and microglia, where they can reduce inflammatory responses. Usually, when we talk about the effects of cannabis, we are talking about what happens when THC binds to the CB_1 receptors in the spinal cord and brain. It is here where the effects of THC are noticed by the person using cannabis. The CB_1 receptors are also responsible for increasing appetite, and so if you have ever used cannabis and got the serious munchies, you can thank this little CB_1 receptor. Interestingly, when you block CB_1, you will not feel hungry even if you use cannabis, and this mechanism has been exploited to develop the drug *rimonabant* to help fight obesity.

Back to the question at hand and what the research tells us. Overall is it good, bad or somewhere in between? The answer is actually somewhere in between. There has been a vast amount of research done on cannabis and how it affects the brain, but the problem is that it can be tough to compare the results from different studies against each other. They use different age groups, types or numbers of people. Some of these will have previously used drugs, and some will have never touched any in their lives. This means that it is difficult to get a concrete answer, and naturally, every scientist thinks that it is their research findings that are the correct ones. This is why the answer can be a little hazy, depending on where you look. However, what is generally agreed upon is that smoking cannabis at a young age is a bad thing. It lowers the brain's learning and memory processes and correlates with the chance of developing symptoms of psychosis (a detachment from reality), such as hallucinations and delusions, in adult life.[2] That said, there is even some debate here, particularly around whether people develop symptoms and then decide to self-medicate, or if cannabis directly leads to psychosis.

This link between cannabis and psychosis is not all down to age though, because there is also a genetic component, meaning that your DNA can make you more susceptible to experiencing severe symptoms from cannabis. Because cannabis, and all drugs of abuse, act on the dopamine system, people with a genetic alteration to one of the dopamine receptors are five times more likely to develop psychosis.[3] Although not entirely understood, the brain's dopamine pathways (the *mesolimbic* and *mesocortical* pathways for those of you who are interested) are responsible for many symptoms experienced during schizophrenia, including hallucinations. Not wanting to break with the tradition of conflicting results, there remains an ongoing discussion about how much dopamine is released in the brain when consuming cannabis, and how influential it is for causing symptoms.

The effects of cannabis use don't end there. Scientists have shown how hard the brain needs to work to keep attention levels normal while someone is taking cannabis (this may come as little surprise). Cannabis use increases the activity in our brain's attention areas and reduces the activity in the memory areas when we are asked to perform a task.[4] Increased brain activity might sound like it is a good thing, but it demonstrates how much strain cannabis puts on the brain. It needs to work harder to maintain the same level of concentration (typically less than normal) compared with a person who is not under the influence of any drugs.

MAYBE CANNABIS IS A TRICKY ONE, BUT CANNABIDIOL IS GOOD FOR ME, RIGHT?

Cannabis does have benefits to it, speaking strictly from a neuroscience point of view, of course, *cough, cough*. Ever since the 1970s and 1980s, scientists have insisted that cannabis could be used to help people suffering from anxiety and depression, along with many types of pain. We now understand that many of the benefits are a result of the *cannabidiol* found within the cannabis plant.

Cannabidiol, or CBD, makes up approximately 20-40% of cannabis extracts, and is associated with many of its benefits, such as anti-inflammatory effects, improving sleep and limiting the severity of seizures.[5] Numerous studies and clinical trials have also proven how useful CBD can be for people suffering from different types of pain. Nerve injuries that cause pain (neuropathic pain), cancer pain and even pain associated with neurological disorders (e.g. multiple sclerosis, which is characterised by brain inflammation) have all been shown to be reduced when using CBD.

One of the big areas where CBD offers a benefit is emotional regulation in mood disorders. CBD can reduce anxiety by altering the signals between the brain's fear and logic centres (signals going from the amygdala to both the PFC and ACC). When CBD gets to your brain, it acts a little like the teacher telling the naughty kids to stop talking. These brain areas now have to limit their conversation, with the fear centre being quiet and the logical areas taking over. This causes an alteration in how the brain interprets fear, downplaying it from a severe event to a scary but safe observation. Recent studies have shown that there could be a benefit of CBD in social anxiety disorder, too.[6] Because CBD seems to quiet the emotional parts of our brain, particularly our own perception of how we are behaving, in stressful situations like public speaking our brain is less bothered by how the audience feels towards us, and thus we experience lower levels of anxiety.[7]

This is significant when we also consider the potential use of CBD in people suffering from fear-related behaviours, such as *post-traumatic stress disorder* (PTSD). The effect of CBD is so impressive that the body already creates its own version called *anandamide*. It is released from our brain cells in order to dampen down other types of brain signals. When looking at the brain of people suffering from PTSD, we see that they have less anandamide, meaning there is the potential for a larger activation of the stress and fear pathways because the brain can't limit those messages. That is why, in small doses, cannabis can sometimes improve symptoms of PTSD.

It's true that the science behind some of the specific scenarios by which cannabis can directly affect the brain is a little scattered. Overall, when taken under medical supervision as an adult, there are many positive effects on the brain, and it can help people who cannot find any relief in other therapies.

WHY DO WE SEEM TO CLICK WITH SOME PEOPLE AND BECOME INSTANT FRIENDS?

Have you ever met a new person and managed to strike up a conversation with them that felt like you had known each other for years? No? Me neither! But this does happen to some of the more social butterflies amongst us. Considering all of the people we interact with on a daily basis, be it in work, school or just out and about, sometimes we meet someone and we just 'click'. The conversation flows naturally, you are both interested in the same things, and you can almost predict what the other is about to say.

Social psychology explains a lot about this process, and that it occurs from a combination of things like our body language, facial expressions, eye contact and, of course, a general interest in the person. All of this is correct, but neuroscientists have never been able to observe this happening in the brain. Until now!

A few years ago, a research team led by neuroscientist Miguel Nicolelis managed to get a good look at the brain as this social connection was happening and revealed what is really going on.[8] As it turns out, our brains change their activity in such a way as to create brain waves that match the other person's brain. This effect is called *coupling*. It explains how our brain synchronises with other people in social situations, explaining why we click with some people better than others. When this synchronisation occurs between two people, a look

21

inside their head would reveal a brain that is expertly mirroring social cues like body language and facial expressions, creating similar patterns of brain signals. This would make the conversation and interaction much more enjoyable, provided that you had a healthy interest already.

The next time people say they are on the same wavelength as you, they may be right!

The research team investigating this brain synchronisation has plans to observe sports teams, musicians, audiences and other groups performing the same task to see how the synchronisation of all the brains helps people work together for a shared experience.

HOW CAN YOU CREATE THIS SYNCHRONISATION WITH SOMEONE?

The brain will synchronise with others based on social cues such as body language, and MRI scans reveal just how important eye contact is in helping our brains to synchronise. Eye contact generates a much stronger level of brain activation than almost any other social cue.[9] We know this is the case because merely looking at a picture of an eye doesn't stimulate the brain in the same way – it really needs the social element.

The synchronisation can also happen in many other ways that you might expect. Simple verbal communication, like having a great conversation, will result in a level of brain synchronisation with the person you are talking with. The brain will synchronise by observing non-verbal communication such as facial expression and hand gestures, although the other person must share an identical emotional response to what you say (they have to care about what you are saying). The synchronisation is lost when the person speaks a language that you don't understand.

I HAVE HEARD THAT MIRROR NEURONS CAN HELP IN SOCIAL SITUATIONS, BUT WHAT ARE THEY?

The coupling effect between two brains is still being investigated, but it is likely to be a feature of how our *mirror neurons* work. Mirror neurons have spent their time in neuroscience as something akin to a tooth fairy. There is evidence of their existence (sadly, no tooth-fairy money though), but for a long time, many scientists doubted their existence, and even today, there is debate as to what they actually do.

Mirror neurons were first discovered in 1992, when Italian researchers found that the brain of a macaque monkey would become active, in the *premotor cortex*, when it performed a motor task, like grabbing an object or eating food.[10] A little obvious, but there is more. What was surprising was that the same area of the brain would become active simply through it watching another monkey grab the same object. It is almost as if the brain was acting out the task through some psychic connection (it wasn't). The term mirror neurons was introduced to describe the neurons that became more active when watching something rather than actually doing the same thing yourself. Neuroscientists were quick to suggest that these mirror neurons would be necessary for learning how to do something by watching how others do it. Shortly after, the search for these mysterious mirror neurons in humans began.

For a time, many scientists didn't believe they existed in humans and that we had evolved past the stage where we would need them (probably a little arrogant of us). Eventually, we started to look at brain activity in people who watched others perform a task. Functional MRI (fMRI) scans revealed the same mirror neurons in people as they saw in the monkeys, but the search didn't stop there. They have since been discovered in lots of places, including the cerebellum (fine motor skills), visual cortex (seeing things) and the limbic system (emotions).[11]

So, why do we see them in other areas of the brain? Although some scientists are still not convinced, many, myself included, believe they are involved in observing other people's facial expressions and emotions, in order to relay empathy and other social behaviours. They are likely to be involved in how our brain synchronises with others during social interactions, particularly by mirroring positive emotions like smiling and laughing, making for a better social connection. It is this involvement that will explain how we click with other people and how easily we synchronise our brain activity. If the mirror neurons of both brains are aware of the many social cues like eye contact, then there will be a higher probability that the brains will experience the coupling effect, and we will have a best friend for life.

The involvement of mirror neurons in emotional responses led some to speculate that autism disorder, where a person has difficulty relating to others, may result from damaged or underdeveloped mirror neurons.[12] Suppose a person can't interpret other people's facial expressions and social behaviours. In that case, we can't expect the brain to know how to formulate its own social behaviours – but we need more studies to really understand this better.

We still haven't seen a mirror neuron up close. We generally rely on brain scans such as from fMRI, and so many questions remain unanswered. Are they somehow different from other neurons in their shape, connections or receptors? Are they normal neurons that also function as mirror neurons? When do they develop, and do we lose them with age? The mystery continues.

Does learning extra languages impact other brain functions and memory?

Those of you who have struggled your way through the seemingly endless array of new words and grammatical rules to learn a new language can attest to how hard your brain needs to work to remember it all. It turns out that because the brain is working overtime to learn a foreign language, it needs to improve its connections between brain regions, and it starts to create extra brain cells just to keep up with this new world you have thrown at it.

Using language is a very complex process involving formulating sentences, understanding the meaning and context, reading, writing, grammatical rules and listening to sounds, and the brain organises all of these processes into a fluent conversation for when we need it. There are areas dedicated to language, such as *Broca's area*, which produces speech and sentence structures so we communicate effectively. *Wernicke's area* is an important region for understanding the meaning behind the words, and the *angular gyrus* helps us to grasp the concepts behind the words themselves. These areas are scattered throughout the middle of the brain, and work with many others to enable us to talk freely and express our inner thoughts.

However, several regions in the brain are altered in people who can speak another language. Areas in the frontal lobe, behind your forehead (such as the PFC and ACC), and an area called the *supramarginal gyri* all play an important role in language. They link words with their meaning and context. The language centres will connect with memory regions to pick out the potential words, but it is the frontal lobe that will check them, making sure they fit with whichever idea you wish to convey. As someone who is trying to learn other languages (emphasis on the trying part), I often find myself thinking hard about what I would like to say. When this happens, my brain seems to believe that it is a great time for apparently random words to pop into my head – making me slow to decide on what to say and probably making me look silly in the process. This is actually my brain's way of trying to match the correct word with the correct context for what I need – a process that gives my brain a real workout.

The PFC and ACC work hard in the brain when speaking a second language. They continuously monitor what you are saying and help you to choose the correct words at the right time, and in your preferred language. This is why brain scans will show these areas as enlarged and with better connectivity to regions around them in those who speak more than one language. MRI scans reveal that bilingual brains (those speaking two languages) have increased grey and white matter, which is a fancy way of saying the brain has more neurons. They work hard, and so they need extra support. The brain tries to couple these new words with new meanings, which is why it needs a greater number of neurons and connections (remember, these connections are synapses that are going to other neurons to help the brain form memories and associations).

What all this means is that the brains of bilingual people are a little different, and this also shows when people are asked to perform cognitive tasks. People who speak a second language generally do better with higher cognitive functions like task-switching (basically, this is what we think of as multitasking), and appear to have better social skills and empathy towards others.[13] This is most likely because putting yourself in vulnerable positions to learn something new helps you to appreciate the difficulties that it takes to master a skill. It is also likely to be linked with the idea that as you expose yourself to new cultures and traditions, it helps to build better insight, empathy and social skills. It is not yet known if learning more than two languages has an even greater impact, but it wouldn't be surprising to see additional improvements in those who learn multiple languages.

LANGUAGE AND AGE

For a long time, it was considered very unlikely for a person to learn a language as an adult or at least to be any good at it. It was generally accepted that it must be learned at a very young age, when the brain is still developing (even though the brain continues to develop into your mid-late 20s). We now understand that is simply not true and you can be an excellent student of languages, or anything for that matter, at any age. The benefit to learning as a child is that you have the immersive environment and a family who encourage you to learn every day. Even the most dedicated adult learner would find a full-immersion into a new language a little intense. But the truth is the brain is capable of learning even once it is a fully developed adult brain.

It may be worth learning a language as an adult, if not for the experiences it may bring, then for its ability to slow down the brain's ageing and hold off things like Alzheimer's disease. When this type of neurodegeneration occurs in bilingual people, the neurons still get damaged and lose some function just like any other brain, but the symptoms (things like forgetfulness) are much less severe. It has been estimated that learning additional languages can delay some of the symptoms by at least five years.[14] What's more, extra languages can also help people achieve a better outcome after suffering a stroke, especially in their attention levels and memory.[15] Presumably, the symptoms are less severe because the brain has more neurons (and connections) in the memory regions of the temporal lobe, and so the brain can preserve more function when damage does occur.

If ever you needed a reason to learn a new language, now you have one. Vamonos!

WHY DO WE GET ADDICTED TO THINGS?

What is addiction? When scientists talk about addiction, it generally means that someone is compulsively looking for and taking drugs,[a] regardless of any negative consequences that come from doing so. It is a long-term disorder that is heavily influenced by our emotions and experiences, resulting in a very serious condition. The processes that lead to addiction and ultimately, tolerance (where the body gets used to the drugs) are really complex, but the following pages will give a good overview of some of the major things that happen. It is important to remember that addiction involves many different parts of our brain, social cues, and lifestyle habits.

From the brain's point of view, we need certain things as human beings to keep us going, such as food, water, a partner and security. When we get those things, our brain can reinforce these behaviours by releasing dopamine to make us feel good. In a way, it entices us by making us feel great when we get something that is essential, and because we like feeling good, we want to do it again. Something similar happens when we find something unique and exciting, presumably because finding something new could be useful to us from an evolutionary standpoint. This dopamine system is what neuroscientists call the *reward pathway*. Unfortunately, the

[a] We can be addicted to almost anything, from coffee, drugs, nicotine and alcohol to gambling and social media. As long as we appear to gain some benefit from it, the brain will want more.

30

reward pathway can be exploited by drugs, ultimately leading to addiction.

Dopamine

You may have heard dopamine mentioned before, often called the 'feel-good' chemical. When we take drugs open to abuse (cocaine, opiates, alcohol, nicotine, amphetamines, etc.) dopamine is released from specific neurons in the brain, causing us to feel good and euphoric, and ultimately motivating us to do it again. This works because our brain makes its decisions based on past experiences and how we felt during them. When the brain thinks about doing 'recreational' drugs again, it will start to talk to other parts of the brain in the memory, emotional and prediction areas.

Although we understand a lot about addiction, the precise way dopamine influences our emotions is not perfectly clear. What we do know is that the brain loves taking drugs. Up to 10 times the amount of dopamine can be released from drugs of abuse compared with natural rewards like food. Fun fact – this might not be true in every instance, because in some people food may be capable of releasing extra dopamine, leading some scientists to believe it could be involved in eating disorders and obesity.[16]

OK, so now that we know what dopamine does, let's put on the lab coat and hit you with some major science. The main dopamine areas within the brain are found in the midbrain structures just above the ears, called the *ventral tegmental area* and *substantia nigra*, or the VTA and SN for short. The VTA projects long neurons to other areas of the brain, such as the nearby *nucleus accumbens*,[b] a structure that is crucial in the brain's reward system. It is the neurons here that are stimulated by drugs and release lots of dopamine. All drugs of abuse increase dopamine like this, which essentially hardwires the brain to find more drugs.

Think about when you train a dog. When the dog does something you like, such as 'sit' or 'bring me a cold beer', you give a treat to reinforce that behaviour. Our brain does the same thing, except in this scenario, we are the dog, and dopamine is our treat.

THE WHOLE BRAIN

So, we take drugs, dopamine gets released, and then what? Addiction is a combination of actions with one goal in sight – get more drugs. Following the initial drug-seeking behaviour, other parts of the brain start to get involved. Dopamine is essentially the gateway into the addiction, but our addicted brain needs to find a way to change the drug-seeking behaviour from voluntary to compulsive (taking us into classic addiction territory).

The hippocampus and amygdala get recruited quite early on. They are the big coordinators of memory and emotions and produce very powerful feelings towards drug-taking that become extremely difficult to overcome. Essentially, in order to tell the brain why the drugs are a good idea in the first place, these two areas like to reminisce about how good it felt when

[b] The nucleus accumbens fits into what is called the mesolimbic pathway (meso = middle, limbic = border, which just describes the location in our brain). Have you ever experienced euphoria from drugs? Brain scans tell us this happens because the mesolimbic reward pathway is running in overdrive and extremely active, creating that sense of happiness.

we used drugs the last time, giving it a 5-star review, so we want to use them again. This is how drug-induced dopamine creates what is called conditioned learning, meaning the brain learns that seeking out drugs is a good thing, and over time, makes it appear more meaningful than it really is, eventually prioritising drugs.

The frontal lobe, specifically the prefrontal cortex (PFC) and anterior cingulate cortex (ACC), are responsible for a lot of our cognitive control and are involved in our thoughts about how great the next drugs will be. Reinforced by the hippocampus and amygdala's backing, they create a kind of report about why it is a good idea to take more drugs, and submit it to the big boss, the *orbitofrontal cortex* (OFC). This is a small area that sits behind the eyes at the front of the brain, and makes important decisions. The OFC has the final say about what we should do next, and combines all of the previous messages together, making the decision to use drugs again.

Through all of these mechanisms, the drugs trick the brain, including the OFC, into making poor decisions. Addiction, in simple terms, is the brain's memories and desires being ramped up, while the expertise and judgement of the OFC are being turned down. The drugs make the brain think it continuously needs more of them.

The science behind the dopamine reward system stems from outstanding research by Wolfram Schultz, who looked at the electrical signals from dopamine neurons in the 1990s and found that the brain will eventually learn to predict that dopamine will be released when recreational drugs are ingested.[17] When this happens, we will ultimately need more of the drug next time to produce the same dopamine high which is how the brain builds up a tolerance.

When we understand how drugs exert such a powerful influence on the brain, it is easy to see how anyone can be vulnerable to addiction (and not just from drugs). It becomes less about what we personally may want, and more about how our brain compels us to prioritise drugs over everything else and takes away our ability to make better decisions.

CAN I BE ADDICTED TO SOMETHING GOOD?

Now that we know a little more about the reward pathway, we can actually use it to our advantage. For example, because the brain responds really well to experiences that are better than we expected them to be, we can create our own rewards. Imagine winning £20 on the lottery. It feels great not only because you have the extra money, but because in reality, you didn't genuinely expect to win. In some way, it can feel like a surprise win.

So, if you need to learn a new language (because we now know how much helps the brain), give yourself rewards along the way. Maybe have a box of treats where you pick one at random, perhaps a piece of chocolate, a walk outside or bungee jump from a tall bridge. This will surprise your brain and keep things fresh and exciting. If you work extra hard, treat yourself with an even better reward. Eventually, your brain will give you dopamine just for thinking about the reward, and you will also feel great for eating the delicious chocolate. Keep this up and what happens next, as neuroscience tells us, is that you will start to feel great not just from the reward but from the stimulus to the reward (the studying). You literally feel good from working hard. In case you are interested, scientists have also shown that money works as a reward in our brains.[18] This may sound obvious, but from an evolutionary standpoint, it was quite an unexpected finding.

IS THERE SUCH A THING AS AN ADDICTIVE PERSONALITY?

There may be a link between drug abuse and our DNA, but it is still unclear. The data tell us that addiction can, to some degree, be inherited; however technically, the genetic changes that lead to addiction are not thought of as something that is carried across generations. Instead, they likely contribute to our individual personality traits, which, when coupled with lifestyle, may encourage addiction in a more predictable way.[19] Addiction for hallucinogens is less likely to be the result of DNA, compared with cocaine, for example. It is very difficult to understand the genetic component in a meaningful way because not everyone who uses drugs will become addicted. In addition, the brain is susceptible to two types of influence, often called nature versus nurture. In other words, our DNA (nature) encodes our cells and tells them how to act, but so can our lifestyle (nurture) or the interaction between the two. The body adapts and changes can occur even after the DNA instructions have been decoded, termed epigenetic changes.

Think about smoking cigarettes. We all know the risks behind smoking, which leads to cancer. The chemicals from smoking change some of the processes in our body and increase the likelihood of developing cancer. This is a lifestyle influence (the nurture part) that is not necessarily hardwired into our DNA (though some people may be more susceptible). For drug addiction, the drugs themselves can cause alterations in our brain cells. Drugs turn genes on or off (genes are short sequences of DNA that code for specific things). These gene changes will alter the production of proteins within the neurons, which in turn can change how our body responds to the drugs. This has been consistently shown in the nucleus accumbens, a region involved in the dopamine reward pathway.

A lot of the DNA changes that have been linked with addiction revolve around the function of neurotransmitters such as dopamine and serotonin.[c] As we have seen, the neurotransmitter levels play a vital role in addiction pathways, and coupled to behavioural and emotional influences from our lifestyle may lead to an alteration in the precise control of the neurotransmitters. This can influence the likelihood of addiction and behaviours like impulsivity.

Overall, there is a genetic component to drug addiction but scientists are starting to understand that it is more about how the drug reacts to us personally, than simply what our DNA says. Ultimately, it comes down to a huge number of lifestyle factors that we can try our best to control.

WHY DO PEOPLE GO THROUGH WITHDRAWAL?

Now we know about how addiction starts – with increased dopamine activating other regions to keep the addiction going – why do people go through a withdrawal phase when they stop taking drugs?

Withdrawal is a combination of many different processes, including tolerance and physical dependence. During drug abuse, the human body will always adapt to oppose a change

[c] Genes for monoamine oxidase A (MAOA), the serotonin transporter (SLC6A4) and the corticotrophin-releasing hormone receptor 1 gene. COMT (catechol-O-methyltransferase) metabolises dopamine, noradrenaline and other catecholamines. A slight variation of the COMT gene giving rise to Met158 alleles and Val158 alleles is linked to an increased risk of methamphetamine and nicotine addiction.

and maintain a balance, a *homeostasis*. Therefore, when high levels of dopamine and other neurotransmitters are consistently experienced by the brain, it tries to adapt itself in an attempt to reduce these levels to a more manageable amount.[d]

To do this, the neuron can change by decreasing the number of receptors it has that the drug can bind to. This helps to control the amount of activation a neuron gets. By having fewer receptors, the drugs will have a more difficult time finding them and activating the neuron. This is why chronic drug users need more drug over time because the brain gets used to the drugs.

The problem is that the brain expects high levels of drugs, and with it, the release of neurotransmitters like dopamine, serotonin, and noradrenaline. In fact, the brain is so good at expecting the drug, it can predict when it thinks you are about to take drugs (for example, it can tell the heart to slow down if it thinks the drugs will increase the heart rate). At this point, the brain has a physical dependence on the drug meaning that the brain works the way that it does because it is *expecting* the drug, and dependent on its arrival.

When an addicted person suddenly stops taking the drugs, however, the dopamine pathways are not stimulated anymore, and the brain is caught off guard. Because the brain is trying to keep a homeostasis, the brain activation will be at a low level in preparation for drugs. When the drugs don't arrive, it results in physical symptoms of withdrawal.

Think of it like you are at a concert and your favourite band is playing on stage. They are famous, having played for

---

[d] Non-neuronal cells such as astrocytes can collect dopamine from the synapse. Cellular changes in the dopamine neurons themselves can up-regulate autoreceptors, which bind their own dopamine to form a feedback loop.

years, and are expecting bigger crowds because of it (tolerance). Eventually, the band pay for the biggest arena in the country because they expect to have sell-out crowds each time (dependence). When a person stops taking the drugs (there will be no fans) the band is left in a gigantic arena with only a few people in the back, and the sound of crickets.

This physical dependence occurs because the band depend on the crowd in order to motivate them to play and pay for the expensive venue costs. Without it, the band find themselves with a low mood, irritability, and a lack of motivation to play. Similar to what we see in people struggling with drug withdrawal.

Things are a little different with drug withdrawal from opioids. These drugs block receptors (instead of activating them), particularly in an area of the brainstem called the *locus coeruleus* (L.C.). This area sends out noradrenaline to regulate things like breathing, blood pressure, and our attention levels. With the opioids blocking the receptors, the L.C. has to work harder to regulate these processes (I mean, we need to breathe, right?) by sending out more noradrenaline. Like if the entrances to the concert were blocked and the fans couldn't enter to hear the band play. The band would just crank up the volume so everyone could hear, even the people stuck outside. This is what the L.C. does. It cranks up the noradrenaline. When the opioids stop, the L.C. keeps sending out lots of noradrenaline (or the band keep on playing), causing an overactivation, resulting in anxiety, muscle cramps, and gastrointestinal problems. In addition, it also results in low dopamine because opioids interact with the dopamine reward pathway mentioned earlier.

Nevertheless, the brain does eventually notice what is going on, and works to rebalance the receptor levels over the following weeks or months (and many other changes). In the meantime, the frontal cortex, the area heavily involved in decision-making, is working overtime to give us cravings, making it more likely that we relapse into drug-seeking behaviours. The frontal cortex is so intensely involved in these cravings that blocking the neurotransmitter released from this area, glutamate, reduces relapse rates.[e] Relapse also comes from the same cues that cause the addiction in the first place, and from a desire to stop the symptoms of withdrawal. These processes make it difficult to stop an addiction.

[e] Blocking glutamate inhibits the reward circuit in our brains and reinforces the negative emotions and thoughts associated with any withdrawal (through the nucleus accumbens and amygdala connections). Serotonin and GABA (gamma aminobutyric acid) also play a crucial role in withdrawal circuits in the brain.

Why Do We Get Memory Loss When We Hit Our Head?

It has been the plot of more TV shows and movies than I would care to name, but is it actually true that a blow to the head makes someone forget recent memories, and even who they are?

Spoiler alert, the latter, not really. Trauma to the head, and therefore the brain, rarely makes a person forget who they are. It might make a good TV drama, but it doesn't really resemble real life. Despite a TV show's creative licence, it is common to have memory loss surrounding the events that occurred close to the time of the head injury, however.

Typically, when we talk about a *traumatic brain injury* or TBI, there will be some level of memory loss. Losing memories is one of the most common complaints people have, and they can be slow to come back. More often than not, the memories surrounding the time of the injury never return.

This type of memory loss is called *retrograde amnesia* and typically involves being unable to remember what happened in the 6–24 hours before the injury. When the head is injured, the brain suffers a physical shock inside the skull, resulting in the death of brain cells and slowing down of the neuronal processes that result in long-term memory formation. The cell death itself is largely the product of inflammation in the brain. This is a secondary response to the original TBI. The inflammation occurs due to the billions of *microglial cells*, which amongst other things, act as the immune cells of the brain. The inflammation attacks neurons and disrupts the processes that the brain needs to do its job. MRI scans of TBI resulting in amnesia will show damage to the temporal lobe and parts of the PFC, both of which are important for creating and storing memories.[20]

People suffering from this type of brain injury have also been shown, in some instances, to struggle with creating new memories (*anterograde amnesia*), forgetting appointments and new people they meet. Some neuroscientists believe that our non-declarative memory, which is our subconscious memory for learning skills and habits, can also be damaged. This would mean that people may struggle to reach the level of skill they had at sports, bike riding or painting, for example, all of which involve other areas of your brain, like the cerebellum at the back of the head. Despite the theory, which at this stage is mostly anecdotal, research hasn't been able to prove this happens on a regular basis.[21]

So, hitting your head can cause a small amount of brain damage that stops you creating long-term memories. Although you may never fully remember the recent memories, the brain does recover, and you can start making happy memories again in no time.

What is Sleep, and Why Do We Do It?

Although it may seem natural and easy for us to do (for some more than others), sleep is a complex relationship between neurons in different parts of the brain and their intricate release of chemicals called neurotransmitters. The reason we sleep is still argued by scientists today, but it is generally accepted that it is used as a time for our brains to organise and process the information and emotions that we experienced during the day, and to replenish neurotransmitters ready for the next day.

The time that we fall asleep, and for how long, is controlled by our brain's internal clock. This clock sits inside the hypothalamus in a place called the *suprachiasmatic nucleus* (SCN – a much easier way to say it). It synchronises our sleep and wake cycle but also many other things, like our temperature and feeding times, and has a lot of control over our daily regulation of genes and proteins. A cycle of regulation that takes, you guessed it, 24 hours. For now, though, we can just focus on the sleep part.

The brain cells in the SCN receive messages from our eyes about the amount of daylight around us. During the day, when the SCN receives those messages, it knows to inhibit the production of the hormone melatonin by the *pineal gland* (a tiny area just above the ear). When there is no daylight, melatonin is produced and released, telling our brain that night time is on the way. We have other cues, like food or activity, which means we don't suddenly fall asleep as soon as the sun goes down. When our brain knows that it's time for bed, the melatonin starts to increase and peaks around two hours later.

Have you ever woken up at a regular time in the morning without the need for an alarm clock? The time we wake up is also dictated by our melatonin levels. So, if you wake up at the same time each morning, it means that your melatonin cycle is perfectly tuned to you.

Our sleep–wake cycle, also called the circadian rhythm, is more important than simply waking up on time. Low quality and duration of sleep can lead to high blood pressure and cardiovascular disease.[22] Even more serious is the link between sleep and Alzheimer's disease: poor regulation of our brain clock can influence symptoms of Alzheimer's disease.[23] What's more, and this is something that scientists are still trying to understand, Alzheimer's disease itself causes changes in sleep patterns, showing that the two are somehow intertwined, and just how vital sleep is to your brain.

So, what happens if you live in a place with lots of light or lots of darkness? Some regions within the Arctic Circle experience months of continuous darkness at a time, but people manage to somehow survive. This supports the view that our brain uses many different cues alongside daylight to control our circadian rhythm, but research does tell us that constant light or darkness can reduce our ability to fight off infection and may be a risk to our health.[24]

WHAT ARE BRAIN WAVES?

Scientists can watch your brain as you sleep, and what they notice is a consistent sequence of brain waves that occur as you fall asleep. Brain waves are patterns of firing for your entire brain rather than just a small number of neurons. It is a sort of singing that your brain does while it is working. Sometimes it is very active, and so the singing is fast and frantic, and sometimes it is sleepy, and the singing slows down to a more mellow jazzy tune. These brain waves can be detected using an EEG (electroencephalogram) headset so that brain activity can be monitored.

When you are awake, and your brain is alert and attentive, it produces low-voltage, but high-frequency waves called beta waves. This is the baseline hum as your brain goes about its daily business. As we try to sleep, our brain firing changes into alpha waves (high frequency, and more regular peaks). Once we become drowsy and start to fall into light sleep (non-rapid eye movement, NREM) the brain begins to sing more softly and calmy, producing its pattern of firing shown as delta waves before falling into a deep sleep. Delta waves (long, slow waves) are also observed when the brain falls into REM sleep (rapid eye movement), but they start to incorporate theta waves when we dream. The delta waves are the slow and gentle jazz song of the night.

REM VS NREM

The NREM and REM types of sleep help scientists to separate the different phases of sleep. They refer to our eye movements during each stage, with the deeper REM sleep given its name due to lots of rapid eye movements as we dream (although we also dream in NREM sleep, we are more likely to remember them if awoken during REM sleep). The two are different, and the brain cycles through them during the night, with typically around 3–5 REM cycles, or about 90 minutes of REM sleep, per night. We are still not entirely sure why we sleep in this way but what we do know is that if you don't get REM sleep, especially over a number of weeks or months, it can have an effect on your mental health.

HOW DOES THE BRAIN GO FROM LIGHT TO DEEP SLEEP?

The brain changes from light to deep sleep with the help of neurotransmitters from the hypothalamus (one of the oldest parts of our brain). The hypothalamus is responsible for a lot of things, like producing hormones, regulating our body (homeostasis) and sleep. Over time, we have found the brain, and in particular the hypothalamus, is very compartmentalised, with many smaller areas within it. Therefore, scientists have given a lot of long names to them all. Be prepared for some serious science words right now.

A lot of this activity is coordinated by a sort of supervisor, making sure that parts of our brain go to sleep when told to do so (there will be no late-night binge-watching around here!). This supervisor, called the VLPO (ventrolateral preoptic nucleus), is located in the front part of the hypothalamus and does what any good supervisor would do – it delegates the job to someone else. I mean, why do all the work if you don't have to, right?

The VLPO tells other brain cells to stop releasing orexins (a type of neurotransmitter called a neuropeptide). This is actually quite smart because the orexins do a lot in our brain. They are our little workhorses. To keep us awake, they make sure that 'awake' neurotransmitters are released (noradrenaline, serotonin, dopamine) to flood the brain and keep us alert. But because the VLPO has reduced the orexins, they can no longer help us stay awake by causing the release of those neurotransmitters, and the balance changes to more of a sleep state. This is what we call NREM sleep.

As I said, these orexins love to work and are not going to be bossed around for long.[a] They find their way to another part of the brain called the *pontine tegmentum*. Here, they tell the brain cells to send out loads of acetylcholine (an important neurotransmitter), and we drift off peacefully into the REM phase, or deep sleep. At the same time, brain cells in a place called the TMN (tuberomammillary nucleus, in the hypothalamus), which releases histamine to keep us awake, start to get a lot quieter. The histamine levels drop, keeping us in REM sleep.

This process can be altered by medications that can change the balance of neurotransmitters and trick our brain into making us feel drowsy. Medications can also do the opposite and make us feel more alert (recreational drugs like cocaine are great at this). Some antidepressant medications increase noradrenaline or serotonin, which can affect the duration of REM sleep. This is something to keep in mind because our brains need REM sleep to process all the information from our day, and as mentioned earlier, we really need REM sleep.

It is important to note here that while the neurotransmitters in our brain are undoubtedly important in the sleep–wake cycle, and especially the transition from light sleep (NREM) to deep sleep (REM), they are not the complete picture. As neuroscientists, we know a lot about sleep and

---

[a] Reducing the orexins now means they have a limited capacity to stimulate neurons in the locus coeruleus. This makes noradrenaline and sends it to a lot of areas in the brain, helping us to be more alert. Preventing the release of noradrenaline from the locus coeruleus has the downstream effect of less serotonin being released from an area in the brainstem called the raphe nucleus.

which areas of the brain remain active while we are sleeping because we can observe different brain waves, memory activation, dreaming, and so on, but there is also a lot that we are yet to comprehend. Simply changing neurotransmitter levels does not explain everything, and so while these changes are necessary for sleep, we still have a lot to learn about why and how we sleep.

INFLUENCE YOUR OWN BRAIN CHEMISTRY

Drugs are not the only thing that can affect our sleep. An area within the hypothalamus called the preoptic anterior hypothalamus (POAH) is sensitive to temperature changes. When we are warm and cosy, or take a hot bath, for example, brain cells here can become activated more easily and help us to feel sleepy by releasing GABA, a neurotransmitter that inhibits neurons. It inhibits parts of our brain that keep us awake, and so we want to sleep. This is most effective around one hour before you wish to fall asleep as it aligns with your natural circadian rhythm. Next time you fall asleep in front of the fire, you know why – that cheeky hypothalamus!

If we fall asleep easily when warm, then it makes sense that we are more awake when we are cold. Actually, the same area in our brain, the POAH, also makes us feel more alert when we are cold. Thousands of years ago, if we were warm and in no danger of freezing to death, it would have been safer to fall asleep and let our guard down. Perhaps this would mean we were close to a fire, which would be essential in keeping roaming predators away while we slept. If the environment was cold, then falling asleep could cause our body temperature to drop, which could be deadly, so our brain would want us to be more alert and active. I don't think nature ever thought we would be relaxing in warm soapy baths, but that's OK – it still works.

IS ANAESTHESIA THE SAME AS SLEEPING?

When we go to the hospital for an operation, we get put to sleep. We wake up after what feels like the briefest of moments, and it's all over (you now have a robotic arm, or whatever the surgery was for). We say that you are put to sleep, but is it really sleep? I am reasonably sure that if someone attempted to perform surgery on me while I was sleeping soundly in my bed, I would wake up screaming, surprised and very confused. It is true that the effects of general anaesthesia are very similar to sleep, but it is such a deep sleep that we cannot be woken.

Although we use general anaesthesia every day in hospitals, and with incredible safety records, we don't really know how they work. We know some of what they do, like how they reduce the activity of the thalamus (an important part in the middle of the brain). The thalamus is essentially a gatekeeper between the body and the brain – if you want to get a message to the brain, you need to go through the thalamus. When we are under general anaesthesia, the thalamus stops information coming from our body (for example, the feeling of pain during surgery) and communicating with other parts of the brain. In this example, it would be the somatosensory cortex in the parietal lobe that makes us feel the pain. Reduced PFC activity also results from general anaesthesia, which is why we are not consciously aware of what is happening (thankfully).

One drug called pentobarbital activates the VLPO (remember, this is in the hypothalamus and causes us to sleep). Pentobarbital also stops the release of histamine in the brain, preventing us from waking. Another general anaesthetic called isofluorane inhibits orexin neurons, our little hard workers involved in sleep. This mechanism is not the only thing happening in the brain, but the truth is that we still don't know exactly why they have such a strong effect on us.

WHAT HAPPENS DURING SLEEP PARALYSIS?

Sleep paralysis (SP) is a strange and often frightening experience that occurs just after falling asleep or before waking up. During SP the body is unable to move, and for some, it can feel like there is pressure on your chest, you are falling, or perhaps worst of all, that there is someone else in the room with you.

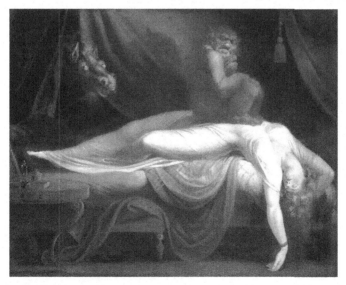

The Nightmare, by Henry Fuseli in 1781, perfectly sums up how scary sleep paralysis can be.

When you sleep, your brainstem stops messages getting to your body that would otherwise make you move. This is so you don't act out your dreams and injure yourself while you sleep. What happens in SP is that the brain is not properly transitioning through the normal stages of sleep – it is somewhere between awake and sleeping. A recent study suggested that the mild hallucinations experienced during SP (for example, someone is opening your bedroom door) may actually be a dream state experienced outside normal sleep.[25] SP occurs because our frontal cortex is more alert than usual while our emotional centre (limbic system) and visual centres (sending messages to the parietal lobe) sense that we may be under threat and cause these dream-like hallucinations.

Although it can be a terrifying experience, we do know that SP correlates with things like jet lag, anxiety and narcolepsy, and so treatment for these conditions may help to lower the frequency of sleep paralysis.

WHAT ARE DREAMS, AND WHY DO WE HAVE THEM?

Now that we know a little more about sleep and why we need so much of it, it's a good time to talk about what happens during sleep. No, I am not talking about cuddling up to your favourite teddy bear – I'm talking about dreams.

Dreams are where we play out an imaginary life where we can fly and visit strange places, or sometimes, encounter creepy Victorian little girls who sing nursery rhymes and giggle in doorways for apparently no reason – our nightmares!

We have all experienced dreams – thoughts and sensations that occur while we sleep – but why we dream has never been fully answered. Throughout the years, there have been many suggestions as to why we dream. Perhaps they are a window into our subconscious mind, or maybe they are a way for our mind to act out our secret desires without social consequences. This was actually demonstrated in one study that recruited people who recently quit nicotine:[26] almost everyone dreamt about smoking in the months after quitting, with dreams becoming more frequent as time went on, presumably as the brain continued to go through withdrawal.

The clearest idea about why we dream is that the brain needs time to process the memories and emotions that we experienced during the day and place them into long-term storage.[27] This makes a lot more sense when we look at the brains of people who are sleeping and see that the hippocampus, the part for memories, and the anterior

51

cingulate cortex, which is involved in assigning emotional context, are particularly active. In fact, on days where we have lots of new experiences, the brain can still be processing this information up to seven nights later. This also partly explains why stressful and emotional events in our lives can significantly affect the quality of our sleep.

One team of scientists demonstrated this by having people play video games for several hours before sleeping.[28] Over 60% of people reported having dreams about the game, suggesting that our short-term memory is particularly active during our dreams.

Furthermore, the dream's events are believed to be a combination of the short-term memories we recently experienced and the long-term memories that our brain thinks are relevant and need to be connected with each other. This supports the view that sleeping and dreaming help to transition our memories from being in short-term storage in the hippocampus to long-term storage all over the brain. This process happens mostly in NREM sleep, and the application of emotional context – how we feel about them – occurs in REM sleep, our deep sleep.

Because some areas of the brain are sleeping, while others are not, we experience this as a strange reality and call it a dream. Interestingly, if we go further into the meaning and symbolism of dreams, we find a more abstract explanation of dreams and a theory that I find particularly interesting.

World-renowned dream specialist Rubin Naiman thinks that we may be looking at dreams entirely the wrong way,[29] and that they are in fact a subset of the thoughts and processes that we experience during the day. They are not particularly special or different to what we encounter during our waking life, and perhaps dreams should be spoken about the same way we talk about the stars at night – they are always there, but we only seem to notice them at night. So, if this is true and we never really stop dreaming, either during the day or night, then why am I not currently writing this book dressed in a pink tutu while sitting on the surface of the Sun? For starters, the pink tutu is currently in the laundry, but the surface of the Sun – well, that is all down to our prefrontal cortex. This is the PFC that we talked about earlier, the area just behind the forehead, which is responsible for logic, planning, attention and generally things that are called executive functions. It's basically the really smart part of the brain. Couple this to the fact that neurotransmitters, the chemicals sent between neurons, are lower than normal and need to be replenished, and you have a recipe for a brain that isn't working entirely as it would be during our waking day.

Try thinking about dreams as if the brain is analysing our daily experiences without much logic. While you sleep, the visual cortex is very much awake. This part of our brain is busy processing the images from the day. Unrestrained, the brain can now think more abstractly and creatively, using imagery and metaphors to express ideas.[30] This is perhaps why scenes and events are often exaggerated during our dreams, yet we don't notice the dream's strangeness (as the prefrontal cortex is sleeping). It is at the point of waking when we recognise how unusual things actually were.

Nightmares

So that may explain dreams, but what about nightmares? Scientists believe that nightmares have an evolutionary purpose and at some point would have been useful for us. They likely evolved to keep us vigilant about dangers or concerns that we may have, so we don't simply brush them off and ignore them. This would have been extremely useful throughout our millions of years of evolution. For example, if our community was attacked there could be potential for it to happen again, or if a lion was seen to be frequently roaming nearby – we would need to keep our thoughts focused on it unless we wanted to be eaten. Dreaming about the stresses and concerns we have is our brain's way of working through the emotions and keeping our attention focused on the danger. As a result, we have nightmares.

Scientists have observed that when people are experiencing nightmares, there is increased brain activity in the amygdala, a key area involved in fear and making fearful events much more memorable. Together with the fact that the prefrontal cortex is generally sleeping too, there is a failure to control and reason with this scary reality, and causing a nightmare.[31]

LUCID DREAMING

There may be potential to harness dreams for our benefit. Lucid dreaming is a fascinating phenomenon, where you are aware of being inside a dream as you are actually dreaming.

Think of it a little like the movie *Inception*, with Leonardo DiCaprio, whereby if you know you are dreaming, you have the potential to make the dream as you want it to be. This phenomenon was first recognised over 40 years ago, and although it has been studied in the decades since, we still can't fully explain why it happens or why some people seem to experience it more than others. Estimates suggest that approximately 50% of people will experience lucid dreams at some point in their lives, 20% of us have them monthly and a small number of people experience them almost every night.[32] What we do know is that the PFC is a lot more active in lucid dreamers. The PFC affects other areas of the brain and starts to increase its signalling to the temporal lobe, which we know is vital in creating and storing our memories. A small study trying to reduce nightmares even found that those capable of lucid dreaming were able to prevent nightmares or limit the distress felt during them.[33]

Lucid dreams occur because of greater connectivity between certain regions of the brain involved in executive functions.[a] In other words, the clever parts of our brain are able to talk to the rest of it more freely during sleep than normal. Although this connectivity has been shown in brain scans, when we talk to people who experience lucid dreams often, they appear just the same as everyone else. Lucid dreamers or ordinary dreamers appear to have the same memory skills, and mindfulness, and demonstrate the same amount of daydreaming as anybody else.

Wouldn't it be interesting if we could take an ordinary dreamer and somehow convert them into a lucid dreamer? Well, because the neurotransmitter acetylcholine is heavily involved in regulating REM sleep and brain signalling in general, it is possible to create lucid dreams by tweaking the amount of acetylcholine in our brains at night. LaBerge and colleagues found that the drug galantamine, which increases acetylcholine, also increases the chance of lucid dreams by over 40%.[35] At this moment, it is unknown if they are identical

---

[a] Connectivity between the temporoparietal regions – specifically the anterior prefrontal cortex–angular gyrus–middle temporal gyrus. This is just a precise way of talking about areas involved in memories, attention, spatial awareness and processing information from our senses about what is around us.[34]

to natural lucid dreams, but it could be a great way to study them in the future with greater predictability.

MAKING DREAMS WORK FOR YOU

What would be a lot of fun would be to try and actually participate in a lucid dream. Could we speak to people inside the dream? Could we ask them what it is like, and use that information to help understand ourselves on a higher level? Is it possible that we could use this technique to talk to our subconscious somehow? Feel free to try this out if you ever experience them!

Would you believe it if you were told there is a device out there to allow you share a lucid dream with another person? Back in 2012, an EEG device attempted to create social dreaming. The idea was that two people would each wear the device (connected to the internet) and when sleeper #1 started to dream, a coloured light bulb would turn on in the bedroom of sleeper #2. With enough practice, the sleeper could notice the light, even while sleeping, make a subtle movement with their eyes or fingers, and the brain activity would be detected and sent back to sleeper #1. They would have their own light bulb that would trigger them to become lucid in each of their dreams. The light would feel similar to hearing your alarm clock go off as you sleep. You would incorporate the noise (or in this case, the light) somehow into your own dream.

By becoming lucid in their own dreams, each sleeper would be aware of the signals. At this stage in the design of the headset you could not really interact with one another, but the idea that you can use your brain waves to send cues to another sleeper, influencing their dream, was a great concept and a notable first step into the area of social dreaming.

If sending messages to the dreamer was the first step, then Konkoly and colleagues recently took the second one.[36] And it was a big step!

Training a group of people to experience lucid dreaming in their sleep labs, the team were able to have two-way communication with the dreamers. They asked the dreamers to answer simple arithmetic, such as 8 − 6, and the dreamer was able to respond back with eye movements (each movement represented a number). They remained dreaming but were able to hear the question as part of their dream. Some heard it as a voice-over, others through their dream-like radio playing in the background.

Although it was difficult for the team to get reproducible results (only around 25% of attempts were successful) some were even able to recall the question upon waking.

This study gives more credit to the idea that we could someday interact with our subconscious dreaming mind gain an insight from our dreams.

One last thought about dreams I would like to share with you is the possibility of using them to your own benefit. Some techniques attempt to utilise dreams as you would any other skill. Have you ever woken up from a dream but forgotten it quickly after? Well, a technique called dream recall may be a solution, whereby shortly after waking, you write down every creative idea you had so that any creativity you encountered can be remembered for when you need it. Famous horror writer Stephen King is well-known for using dreams as a source of creativity for his stories. His book *Dreamcatcher* was actually based on a dream he had about a cabin and hitchhikers.

If you have a particular problem that you need to find a solution to, well then dream incubation is your game! Before falling asleep, it is possible to focus on a problem that you may have. With enough attempts, studies have shown that it is possible to dream about topics of your choosing and use them to target a meaningful area of your life. The mathematical genius Srinivasa Ramanujan is famous for mailing complex mathematical formulas to a University of Cambridge professor in the early 1900s. What makes his story even more incredible is that Ramanujan lived in a small village in India and had no real access to advanced books. From the age of 16 (he was 25 when he mailed his work to Cambridge) he said that formulas would appear before him in dreams, and he was able to develop them when he woke up.

Finally, an intriguing technique called dream prophecy sounds like it would have the most use in our waking life. Who wouldn't like to dream about events before they happen? Maybe you can avoid being late for work or spilling your drink over yourself, or maybe you could concentrate really hard and learn the lottery numbers to win millions. It sounds radical, but there are numerous reports of dreams that apparently play out scenes and interactions that you then experience in your life. Early suggestions tended to be explained as déjà vu, but it is much more likely that the experience is simply a coincidence, considering the thousands of dreams that are not prophetical. It may also be linked to the Baader–Meinhof phenomenon (see Chapter 2), whereby you are more likely to notice these coincidences after being made aware of them, with a strong desire to rely on anything to support your view – like when you think of a friend and they call moments later, yet you tend to forget the times when you think of them without the phone call. Feel free to try it out though!

CAN BRAIN FREEZE KILL YOU?

OK, so as this is a science book, I should at least try and use the correct medical term for brain freeze (also called ice cream headache), which is *sphenopalatine ganglioneuralgia*. You know what? On second thought, that is a bit of a mouthful, so I think we can stick to brain freeze for this part after all. Brain freeze happens when you eat or drink something icy too quickly, causing you to experience a rapid and intense headache, which thankfully goes away just as quickly.

When you quickly change the temperature at the back of your throat near two important arteries, the brain really doesn't like it, because these two arteries are crucial for the brain. The *carotid artery* takes blood to the brain, and the *cerebral artery* distributes it around. The sudden temperature change causes a dramatic increase in the blood flowing through both arteries, which the brain notices.

The pain comes when temperature receptors that line the brain's membrane, the *meninges*, notice the change and send out messages to the brain. The *trigeminal nerve* (the main nerve for the face and head) is activated and causes an intense feeling, which the brain interprets as pain so that you stop whatever it is you're doing (like eating your body weight in ice cream). Brain freeze happens as a way for your body to tell you that the sensation is too intense. The brain likes things to be nice and consistent. It enjoys nothing better than living a boring life where everything is nice, controlled and safe.

Once the mouth and throat warm up, the blood vessels get smaller and the blood flow reverts to normal, which doesn't take long. Although the feeling of brain freeze is not very pleasant and can feel like something serious, it really isn't. Even the strongest headache from brain freeze is simply an intense signal from your brain, and nothing more. There has never been a recorded case of someone dying from it or having any other side effects other than an aversion to ice cream – momentarily, of course.

Interestingly, people who suffer from migraines are more likely to experience brain freeze. Exactly why this happens is not fully understood, but it is being researched in an attempt to find new drugs for migraines.

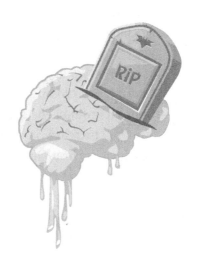

Too dramatic? It can certainly feel like that during brain freeze.

Can Brain Cells Regenerate?

Historically, the brain has been seen as an impressive supercomputer but one that struggles to repair itself and regain function if it becomes damaged. This has never been more obvious than when coming face to face with the seemingly impossible task of repairing brain and spinal cord injuries. Most of the neurons we have after being born will stay with us for the rest of our lives, but despite what you may have heard, the brain does make new neurons, and it can repair itself – to a certain extent.

Before we are even born, the brain cells are dividing at a rapid rate. This process doubles the number of neurons every time. They divide and grow at such a rate that the brain has a surplus of neurons. So many that they slowly and precisely reduce in numbers for much of our childhood. We are born with more neurons than we really need, and over time, we keep only the ones that are useful in helping us to learn and understand the world around us. The surplus is slowly brushed back until we have a lean, mean and efficient brain.

Suppose all of this growth occurs at an early age and nothing more after. In that case, it is easy to see why neuroscientists traditionally believed that the adult brain could not regenerate and grow new brain cells. Even today, there is still an ongoing debate as to the extent of regeneration in adult brains. Brain cell growth, or *neurogenesis*, is a crucial field of research within neuroscience. New scientific techniques that enable scientists to study the living brain using brain scans, or to grow brain cells in the laboratory, have given us unprecedented insight into how neurons grow and develop. What they have revealed is that our brain is continuously making new brain cells. Around 700 every day, to be exact, and this continues well into old age. The oldest person to show neurogenesis is 97![37] That is just in the hippocampus (mostly in an area called the *dentate gyrus*) – we haven't even looked in most other places.

If new brain cells are being made every day, then they should be able to repair themselves after suffering damage, right? The brain and spinal cord can repair themselves within reason, but the problem is that they may never be able to regain all of the connections they once had, resulting in a loss of function. This may be a struggle with movement causing a paralysis, or speech or memory issues. It depends on the area of the brain or spinal cord that is damaged. The human body is smart though, and the brain can learn to rewire itself to adapt to missing connections and look to build them elsewhere. We see this in people who suffer brain trauma, such as a stroke, who manage to regain function, at least partly, if not completely.

What is important to note is that injured neurons can regenerate, and a recent study from a team of researchers in California found that they do this by regressing to a younger state.[38] The neuron, after recognising the damage, will go back to being a baby neuron, when it is capable of regrowing to start a new life, forgetting its adult life when it got injured.[a] For

---

[a] Technically, the changes are seen on a genetic level as it resets a number of genes that promote neuronal changes and regrowth on a transcriptional level, meaning that the RNA changes in order to create new proteins found at an earlier stage in life.

regeneration, the neuron's conditions need to be optimal to promote growth, which is difficult for the body to achieve. Think about when a person gets sick or injured. They go to the hospital to be given medicine and treatments. The environment is constructed in a way as to promote healing and recovery. You wouldn't be expected to make a full recovery if you continued with your daily life as normal, ignoring the injury. This is essentially what research is currently trying to understand. What would that local environment (or hospital setting) look like for damaged neurons? In other words, how do we give the best medicine and treatments for the best chance of brain cell regeneration? This would improve the natural neurogenesis in the brain and improve outcomes from injury.

The hope for the future is that neurons will be able to be grown in a laboratory using the most nurturing conditions (for example, with proteins such as growth factors) and transplanted back to the site of injury. The neurons would then begin to regenerate themselves and the thousands of connections that they had previously made with other neurons. Of course, the brain can do this on its own, but not as efficiently as we would like it to be.

So yes, brain cells can regenerate, but the process is limited, and neuroscience is not yet at the stage where a full recovery is expected in every patient.

So what about disease then? Can neurons recover from diseases like *motor neuron disease* (MND)? Motor neurons send signals from the brain to the muscles all around the body, giving them instructions to move. In MND (also called *amyotrophic lateral sclerosis*, ALS) the motor neurons lose their function, and eventually die. This is primarily due to specific proteins in the neurons not working as they should, leading to a cascade of events that ultimately causes cell death. Other cells, like astrocytes, also become injured and eventually die, which has a big impact on the body's repair mechanisms.

The body can repair motor neurons if they become damaged, from a blunt injury for example, but the real problems occur when there is an underlying disease that causes the neurons to become faulty, and those repair mechanisms can't help.[39] Think of it like building a house. You can have the right blueprints and a team of experienced builders, but if the wrong shaped bricks get delivered, spherical bricks instead of the normal rectangular ones, then the house isn't going to be constructed with the usual stability. Eventually it will crumble, regardless of how good your building team is. This is what happens in MND, and so the regeneration – or building – is very challenging for neuroscientists.

The treatment options for the future are looking more towards stem cell therapy, which will essentially replace the ordered truck of spherical bricks with a truck full of regular bricks, so the house gets built the way it should be.

How are memories encoded in the brain?

When scientists talk about memory, they tend to group it in two different ways. The type of memory that we are all familiar with, where we remember facts and events about our day, is called *declarative memory*. This is a more autobiographical kind of memory – we are conscious of it, and to some extent, have a lot of control over it. The second type of memory, called *non-declarative memory*, is what our brains use without our knowledge, and it is essential for learning new skills and developing habits. Non-declarative memory is also referred to as subconscious memory.

We also have short-term and long-term memory. Our short-term memory applies to anything that we remember for about 30 seconds to a minute and is dictated by our frontal lobes, or in other words, our conscious thoughts about what we are trying to remember. The brain is actually quite limited in its ability to use short-term memory as it can only store between five and nine items of information at any given time.

The hippocampus will eventually be recruited to remember any information for a longer period of time, but if we want to keep something in our long-term memory, so we don't forget it, then the memories are eventually stored throughout the entire brain – a process that can take weeks to complete. In this question, we are going to discover how long-term memories are created and the precise things that our brain cells do in order to recall a memory when you need it.

WHAT ACTUALLY IS A MEMORY?

When we talk about a memory in the brain, what do we really mean? If we think back to a happy childhood memory when we are out playing with our friends, what does that actually look like to our neurons? Is it a group of images, or a short video? If we could look at those neurons (and we can) could we actually see that memory? Technically, it is possible.

Although science has not yet reached the stage where we can decode a memory just by looking at the neuron, there are real changes that happen to each brain cell in order to create a memory. This has been studied a lot, in regards to our long-term memories, in a part of the brain called the hippocampus. Here, there is a very high density of brain cells, and we can study memory formation with a lot more clarity. However, a memory isn't stored like a movie reel of the event – instead, small details about the experience are encoded that we then recreate ourselves every time we remember something. We remake the video from spare parts each time, which is why you will remember it a little differently each time you recall it. In neuroscience, this idea is called a *sparse distributed scheme*, where each memory is encoded by a number of neurons, and those neurons can even be recruited at a later date to help remember something else too.[40] Memories are also dependent on our emotional state, both at the time of the event and when we try to recall it, and so this will play a big role in how we remember something.

As memories are made up of all these tiny details, they are actually created and stored all over our brain, in the brain cell connections that encode our emotional responses, colour, sound, taste and pretty much every other detail you can imagine. The long-term memories are created in a process called long-term potentiation, or LTP for short, which can take anywhere from minutes to weeks to complete. Next, we are going to look at precisely what LTP really looks like to our brain cells.

LONG-TERM MEMORIES IN THE BRAIN

Long-term memories start to be encoded when something happens that causes lots of brain signals, or action potentials, to go to a very specific area all at once. This leads to changes in those neurons, changes that neuroscientists call plasticity. This is why the brain is often referred to as being plastic, because changes can occur throughout our life.

Plasticity alters synapses so that the communication between them is strengthened and made easier and more efficient for the next time. This can happen in a few different ways, but by far the most studied is LTP. Think of a brain cell in terms of a road, a major road going across a city. At the end of the road, there are many exits (synapses) that lead to other smaller roads (dendrites),[a] and eventually, other cities (other neurons). This means that all the exits can be extremely specific to where you want to go (or what you want to remember). If something eventful happens that you want to remember, say you drive to watch a Beyoncé concert, then the exit heading to the stadium will be full of cars, a lot more than usual (in the brain, this would be an increase in action potentials). Because of the grand scale of the concert, the

---

[a] If a neuron is an arm, the dendrites would be the long fingers stretching out to other arms. The synapse would be the fingertips reaching out to touch other fingertips. How romantic!

bottom of this exit (synapse), heading towards the stadium, would lead to a traffic jam.

Therefore, people park their cars and walk to the stadium (the people are neurotransmitters launching themselves toward the next neuron). Once they finally get to the stadium (it takes about 0.0005 seconds) all of the Beyoncé fans find that they need to walk through a narrow gate (AMPA receptor).

Now there is a problem – there are just too many people and too few gates, and so another gate needs to be created (NMDA receptor).[b] With the extra gate now letting people inside, the flow of people is more controlled, but the concert is still very popular (after all, seeing Beyoncé ride an elephant while singing in perfect Korean would be a sold-out event, right?). So, the guy on the gate sends someone up to the road where all the cars are parked, to tell them that it's OK to send more people across because the extra gates are now open.

What is different about this messenger though, is that she doesn't just walk over there like normal. After seeing the crowds, she doesn't want to have to fight her way through. Instead, she grabs a handful of balloons (filled with nitric oxide – if you add an extra nitrogen you will make laughing gas) and floats over to the original road where all the cars are parked. This does actually happen in the neurons, as nitric oxide signals back to the first neuron, acting as a retrograde signaller.

---

[b] When the neurotransmitter glutamate binds to the first receptor (AMPA), or in this scenario, the first gate, it changes the synapse a little. It causes a small change in voltage that releases magnesium, which was sitting in the other gate, or NMDA receptor. Now they are both working and glutamate binds to both.

Now more people get to the stadium to see Beyoncé.[c] This plasticity, or change, can take weeks to be fully developed, but it leaves the brain with a basis for new long-term memories. This whole process is long-term potentiation, and the plasticity refers to the fact that the roads will always have those extra gates prepared, and working more efficiently, the next time you want the memory. The synapse has been permanently changed. You have a new memory!

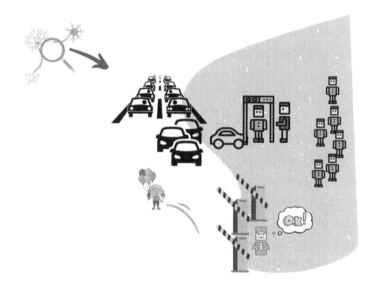

Long-term potentiation is a multistep process but leads to neuronal adaption over time.

[c] Within the neuron, the concert would be equivalent to increased calcium ions, which cause changes inside the neuron to help with creating a memory.

Sometimes, not many people really want to see Beyoncé, and so these changes never quite happen. In this instance, the brain can forget the concert ever happened. This is called long-term depression, or LTD, and it occurs in the cerebellum for things like learning how to walk or ride a bike, because we don't want to remember how to fall down – we only want to keep the memories of when we stay up and are successful. An important note here, however, is that this is only subconscious and not something that we can utilise ourselves – even though I am sure we all wish for the ability to forget the memories we don't want. As far as the science tells us, long-term memories never leave us: they are always stored somewhere, even if they are difficult to remember.

FEAR

Although we talk about the hippocampus as being necessary for creating memories, the reality of the brain is that it is a lot more complex. We are emotional beings, and because of that, we attach emotions to our memories. So, although the temporal lobe (the memory area) is important in making the memories, it has connections to other parts of our brain: parts that will tell us if it is a happy memory, and make us feel good, or a part of our brain that remembers a particular smell (such as perfume, or candles only used at Christmas), which will help trigger memories associated with that stimulus. If you often smell or taste something that brings back a memory associated with it, it's because you are activating those specific brain connections and triggering the entire memory.

We also have the frontal lobes of our brain, which include the prefrontal cortex and anterior cingulate cortex, which act as the chief librarian, looking over the books in the library before you check it out, to make sure it fits with the purpose you want (i.e. gives context and meaning to the memory). In much the same way that we remember happy events in our lives, we can also remember things that have scared us. We essentially learn to be afraid of things that could be dangerous to us. The _amygdala_, a small area at the top of the brainstem, has a big role in our emotions and fear, with connections to many other areas of our brain which help put this fear into context. For example, are we just afraid because we are watching a movie, and in reality, nothing can really hurt us? If that is the case, then our logic centres will explain to the rest of the brain that we don't want this fear to form a debilitating memory (it doesn't always get this right, which can lead to fear and anxiety disorders). In contrast to this, our brain also decides if a scary or dangerous situation, like being attacked in a dark alley, should be remembered. That way, we recognise the danger and develop an appropriate fear of dark alleys at night, thanks to our amygdala, PFC, hippocampus, and others.

A MAN CALLED H.M.

The way that neuroscientists have historically studied the workings of the brain is by observing people after injuries. One way to get a tremendous amount of understanding is to look at what happens when brains are damaged and have lesions. In 1953, a 27-year-old man, named Henry Molaison but referred to by his initials H.M., suffered from severe epilepsy and opted for surgery in an attempt to rid himself of it. The surgery ultimately had tragic consequences. The removal of some of his temporal lobe was so extreme that he lost his ability to form new memories. He could remember the names of friends and family from before the operation, but any new people he met were quickly forgotten. He also lost memories of events that happened to him in the 10 years prior to his surgery.

Interestingly though, if H.M. was asked to briefly remember a string of numbers, he could easily do so, but as soon as he was distracted or started a new task, he would immediately forget. Because of H.M., we now know that the medial temporal lobe is essential for transforming information into long-term memory. Essentially, this is the quiet and polite librarian who organises where the books go so that they can easily be retrieved at a later date. Further studies have shown us that areas in addition to the hippocampus, called the *caudate nucleus* and *putamen*, are really important in learning and memory, and this has also been observed when studying the brains of memory champions (yes, that is a real thing and it is fantastic). Although tragic, we learned a lot from H.M. about how the brain transfers memories into long-term storage and, ironically, he will never be forgotten for this.

IF WE KNOW ALL THIS, CAN WE IMPROVE OUR MEMORY?

How easily do you remember a wedding day, or live sports events, or maybe even a car crash? Do you have to work hard to remember it, or does it come back to you easily? What about a conversation you had with a friend on a random Tuesday a year ago – do you remember what you both talked about?

Some things that happen to us appear to be forever engrained in our memory (for better or for worse) without much effort. There is a reason for that. Our brains love to learn new things and respond well to events with high emotional content that involve many of our other senses (sound, vision, etc.). This would have served an essential function throughout our evolution. If we happened to come across an unexpected body of water that we could drink from, our brain would want to remember it. Or maybe we walked through a dangerous area full of predators that we would need to avoid in the future. Events that happen which activate our emotional responses, like being very excited to see water, are more easily encoded by our brain, ready for a time when the information may be needed. If the brain doesn't think it is novel or particularly interesting (like a conversation you have had a hundred times already), then it will not trigger a substantial response in our neurons, leaving our brain to focus on the more important stuff.

World memory champions use this understanding of neuroscience to their advantage. The brain can remember a sequence of numbers (fewer than 10) for a short period of time before forgetting them. If someone wants to retain them for much longer, they can repeat the numbers over and over with the hope that they will be encoded in the long-term memory. This works because the repeated stimulus will eventually strengthen the synapses, but it is very slow and very boring. Instead, memory champions will associate an imaginary picture, scene or person with a particular number (it also works for things that are not numbers). World memory champion Ryu Song can remember nearly 7,500 binary digits (only 1s and 0s) in just 30 minutes. Due to years of practice, it has been shown that the brains of memory athletes (the official term) change in order to accommodate this superhuman memory. Functional MRI (fMRI) brain scans reveal that the hippocampus and caudate nucleus are both increased in size, and there is improved connectivity between them.[41] This fMRI measurement was so accurate that researchers were able to predict the rankings in the memory championships based purely on brain size.

As the scans were done on people once they had already dedicated years of memory training to their craft, it is unknown if they had superior connectivity (how easily the brain regions talk to each other) or brain sizes prior to becoming memory athletes. However, it is doubtful they did. It is much more likely that they were born with a normal brain, but with the added requirement for their memory tasks, their brain developed this way.

This means that you can improve your own memory with the same techniques that memory champions use. The trick is to imagine something unique, very strange, and that engages other senses like your smell and taste (imagining a foul-smelling troll on horseback could be used for the number 10, for example). Over time, and with practice, these exaggerated scenes and images can help a person remember almost anything, in a matter of seconds. It may seem strange, but for the brain, because it doesn't often see a troll riding a horse, it wants to remember it. Further memory techniques can use locations, such as a house or city that you are familiar with, because they can be filled with many creative images that the brain will recognise more easily.

Try it out for yourself! See if you can remember 7,500 numbers better with fun imagery, rather than just repeating them.

Does a Genius Have a Different Brain?

Are some of us born with a brain that makes us destined to become a world-renowned mathematician or an earth-shattering artist who can reduce any person to tears with a single brush stroke? Are these traits hardwired into our brain from the day we are born, or can they be acquired, adapted and harnessed? Does a genius have a different brain?

When I think of intelligence, I tend to think of a Matt Damon-style character writing equations on a chalkboard, like in the film *Good Will Hunting*. But there are many types of intelligence (current theory puts this at a minimum of nine), such as interpersonal, logical-mathematical and musical. In general, intelligence is dictated by how well the brain is connected to other regions. Let's explore this a little more.

For the purpose of this question, we will discuss logical-mathematical intelligence, which is more along the lines of the traditional view of intelligence and IQ. Neuroscience tends to study intelligence in one of three ways. One way is by examining the brain's structure and function – in essence, does the brain look any different depending on IQ? Another is to search for differences in DNA that could be linked to intelligence. And third is how our environment and life experiences contribute to our intelligence, meaning that if we spend our entire life learning quantum mechanics, there is a good chance that we will improve our IQ.

It is a common myth that people are born smart, and that there is not much you can do after that. If you are not fortunate to be born with the potential for an astronomical IQ, then tough luck. That is not true! But there are differences in the brains of people who have a higher level of intelligence. They do look a little different.

Small bits of brain removed during surgery have shown us that the neurons themselves can have bigger dendrites (the long outstretching arms of the neuron) that branch into more complex pathways with other neurons.[42] What's more is that the frontal and temporal lobe regions of the brain, widely regarded as the source of much of our intelligence, are bigger in people with a higher level of intelligence. Both of these measurements have been correlated with IQ. Put another way, bigger and more complicated brains will make a person smarter.

If that is the case, we would expect the trend to continue and for people with a bigger brain to be the smartest amongst us, right? A research group looked at lots of different studies of brain size and IQ, examining more than 8,000 brains, and did in fact confirm that a bigger brain is one factor contributing to intelligence.[43] However, before we get ahead of ourselves, brain size is only one of any number of variables that contribute to predicting intelligence, not to mention that it is the relative size of the brain compared with the person that is important. The researchers were quick to acknowledge that although it is a factor, in reality, brain size doesn't make a lot of difference – the real impact comes from how well the brain is connected, and how easily it talks to other regions.

This brain connectivity is the secret to many feats of brilliance that the brain pulls off, and as far as neuroscience teaches us, it is the real reason we become more intelligent. MRI scans tell us that when specific brain regions, such as the *anterior insula* and *middle occipital gyrus*,[a] are well connected to the rest of the brain, information is able to flow more freely and efficiently, making our brain just that little bit smarter.[44] This allows for the smart messages to have priority when making their way through the brain – a little like having a genius friend on speed dial while having others in the regular phone book. Brain scans have also revealed that weaker connections between certain other areas that may provide distracting or irrelevant information to the task at hand may also create a more efficient neural network for intelligence.[b]

It is not only this connection to other regions in the brain, but within individual regions too. Imagine it like this. You are talking on the phone with your long-distance relative who is sunbathing on an island somewhere. It's great to catch up, because you need to check to see if they are still coming over for the holidays. Of course, you also need to chat with your immediate family, your parents and siblings, who will be hosting the get-together. Speaking with your parents and siblings is perhaps the most important part of building intelligence. If you can't arrange a holiday meeting in your own home, it won't be much use inviting far-away relatives. When your brain manages to speak to both the close and

[a] The anterior insula is important in things like our self-awareness and decision-making, and the middle occipital gyrus plays an important role in our spatial awareness, i.e. processing your own body and other three-dimensional things in your mind.

[b] Particularly connections with the inferior parietal lobule, involved in the perception of emotions, attention and language. Also the superior frontal gyrus, important in higher cognitive functions and memories, and the temporo-parietal junction, which has many functions linked to our moral guidance, mathematics, perception, attention and social interactions.

distant family clearly and precisely, this has big implications for how intelligence develops.

THE BRAIN OF THE GREATS

That is all fine for most people, but what about the brain of a genius? If we can see differences amongst people in normal scientific studies, then it should be possible to see them in the brain of someone like Albert Einstein, for example.

Einstein's brain has famously been studied for decades (and against his wishes, I might add). Scientists have looked at it in every way imaginable and found a number of striking features. The brain is made up of neurons and a lot of different types of cells called glial cells. They do many different things to assist the neurons, ultimately helping the brain perform at its best. Einstein's brain had many more glial cells throughout, particularly in areas associated with mathematical processing and incorporating and integrating information from different regions of the brain.[c] Combined with a better connection between the two brain hemispheres, it is thought that these differences in Einstein's brain could have been responsible for his famously robust thought experiments and intellectual abilities.

It is worth bearing in mind that in contrast to all of the published data, studying Einstein's brain cannot ever really give us any significant clues into the mind of a genius. For all of the observations, it is still only one brain. For a true understanding, scientists would need to study hundreds of

[c] Two areas showed a greater number of glial cells: the inferior parietal area, which is heavily involved in mathematics, and the angular gyrus, which is part of the parietal cortex and involved in number processing, memory and attention.

genius brains to be able to compare the differences. Many of the studies themselves had several flaws invalidating some of the data. Even the most significant changes that have been observed in Einstein's brain may simply be the result of a lifetime of learning and study, which will result in an improved brain and IQ. So, for all those who suggest that it may offer clues to his genius, others are suggesting that we are asking too much from the research studies.

It is difficult to look back through history and understand what made a person great, but that hasn't stopped another research team from trying. Leonardo da Vinci is widely regarded as one of the most talented people to have ever lived. Famed for his brilliance as an artist, inventor and engineer, exactly what made his brain so spectacular has peaked the curiosity of many for centuries. According to one team of scientists, da Vinci may have had ADHD (attention deficit/hyperactivity disorder), characterised by bouts of procrastination, mind wandering and restlessness.[45]

The group suggests that he was able to positively channel his ADHD to fuel his creativity and allow himself to master his craft, and also hypothesise that he may have had some form of dyslexia, which only added to his originality and overall mystery. We will never know the reality of course, but it does remind us that everyone, regardless of their unique brain, has the potential to be great.

Can you turn your brain into that of a genius? Science tells us that continuously learning and challenging yourself will improve brain volume, connectivity and intelligence, as your brain adapts to the new challenges. According to the neuroscience network theory, everyone has the opportunity to improve their intelligence level, whoever they are. Because intelligence is associated with the structure of the internal brain networks (the immediate family hosting the holiday party in the analogy above), by continuously learning and exposing yourself to new experiences, you will have the best chance to improve your intelligence and IQ, and that it is something that we can all do, even if you don't have a 'genius' brain.

Can the Brain Really Multitask?

When asked, most people feel a great sense of pride in stating that they are incredible multitaskers. They can do two things at once and do them so well that people are in awe of how magnificent they are. But is it all true? Can people really drive while texting, or read a book while writing an email?

Although you may feel you can multitask very well, neuroscience does not back this up. Multitasking has been studied in the laboratory in various ways that allow scientists to record brain activity. What the data show is that the brain is only really capable of giving attention to one thing at a time. The two activities compete for the same brainpower and attention, which really challenges the brain. Because the brain can't do both things at once, it quickly switches its attention between both tasks[46] – a method that scientists call (rather uncreatively) task-switching.

The problem with task-switching is that both tasks are asking the brain for instructions and relevant information about what to do. If we want to read a book and write an email at the same time, we may start to read a chapter, but when we focus back on the email, the brain needs to stop the instructions it had prepared for reading and pull up the blueprints for writing. When we start writing, there is a short delay while our brain adjusts itself from the reading. At the same time, it needs to figure out what information may be relevant, and so our performance drops for each task. Likewise, when our brain switches back to reading, it has to reorganise itself all over again, leading to lower productivity in both reading and writing compared with only doing one of them at a time. Like channel-surfing on a TV. You flick between channels and don't get the full dramatic experience of either TV show.

The reason for this has a lot to do with the executive areas of the brain. The frontal cortex[a] supplies our brain with general cognitive control, meaning that it decides what to give attention to and what information our brains have stored away that it might need to use. It monitors what we do and has the final say in how to apply our attention to the task at hand. Adding extra tasks disrupts this process, which means that our brains cannot multitask.

As we get older, the frontal cortex doesn't work quite as effectively with the rest of our brain. The connectivity between this region and other parts is much lower; for example, between the attention and memory regions. This means that it becomes much more difficult for the brain to task-switch compared with when we were younger.[47]

However, to leave you with some hope, our brains can multitask a little bit, if the tasks are different types of activity. For example, we cannot talk and write effectively at the same time, or listen to a TV show while reading because both tasks require language areas to function at a high level. But our brains can process dual streams of information if the two areas of our brain needed don't overlap. We can listen to music, or an audiobook (say, a particular neuroscience book from a charming Englishman) while performing a motor task

---

[a] The frontoparietal regions involved here include the dlPFC and ACC (dorsolateral prefrontal cortex and anterior cingulate cortex). They are responsible for prioritising our attention to one task and reducing our attention to other, less important tasks.

like running or walking – which is why you don't fall over every time you listen to music on your morning jog. So, if you really want to multitask, try and find creative ways to combine activities that your brain can handle separately.

WHAT IS DEPRESSION, AND DOES IT CHANGE THE BRAIN?

Depression is a debilitating illness with wide-ranging symptoms that vary between people. A short description would be that it is a mood disorder with episodes of negative thoughts and emotions. But in reality, it is a lot more complicated than that. It is a recurrent illness (88% of people experience more than one episode) that creeps into many aspects of life, affecting mood and motivation, sleep and concentration, and eventually leaving people more susceptible to suicidal thoughts.[a] The number of people who suffer from depression each year is shockingly high: it affects around 20% of the population at some point in their lifetime, but usually first appears when people are in their mid-20s to early 30s.[48]

You may have heard a little or a lot about depression already. If you have, it was most likely that it involves an imbalance of a neurotransmitter in the brain called *serotonin*. This idea first arose in the 20th century, when it was discovered that a drug used to treat high blood pressure also helped people with depression-like symptoms. The drug, *reserpine*, appeared to reduce a group of neurotransmitters called monoamines, which include serotonin, dopamine and noradrenaline (AKA norepinephrine for the Americans out there). The theory behind this process is aptly named the

---

[a] For support, there are a number of websites that can offer their services, such as depressionuk.org in the UK, adaa.org in the USA and mdsc.ca in Canada.

monoamine hypothesis. While it is true that reduced levels of monoamines, particularly serotonin, are found in the brain during depression, increasing them during the treatment of depression doesn't always yield great results. The hypothesis that low serotonin causes depression is far from perfect, but it has remained a popular explanation partly because many drugs that increase serotonin can be effective in patients.[b] All antidepressant medications on the market today increase at least one of these monoamines, but the theory remains complicated by the evidence that many treatments take a long time to show any benefit, and around 30% of people don't seem to respond at all.

There is a glimmer of hope. Recently, a new drug, esketamine, was approved for use in depression, and it works especially well in people who don't benefit from normal antidepressants. It starts to work in only two hours and can significantly reduce severe symptoms including suicidal thoughts. It is particularly interesting because it works by a completely different way to other anti-depressants by altering how the neurotransmitter glutamate affects certain pathways in the brain, ultimately increasing brain-derived neurotrophic factor, a protein that helps neurons to grow, and is something which we will discuss below in more detail.

Pharmaceutical drugs are not the only way that scientists are trying to treat depression. In the search for better ways to treat people who do not benefit from traditional therapies, the

[b] When neurotransmitters such as serotonin are released into the synapse, there are receptors on the surface of the neurons that absorb the excess. This is so the neuron receives a rapid signal and isn't in a state of constant activation due to any leftover neurotransmitters floating around. These reuptake receptors are blocked by drugs called selective serotonin reuptake inhibitors (SSRIs). With the drugs, there is now more serotonin at the synapse, which is critical when the levels are low to begin with.

psychedelic drug *psilocybin*, has been tested with great success. For years, there have been suggestions that this hallucinogen can be effective in treating things like addiction, anxiety, depression, and even assisting in meditation. Recently, a small clinical trial proved that psilocybin was effective in both depression and anxiety, likely a result of increasing serotonin and glutamate in the brain.[49] Further studies will be needed with greater numbers, but the early data is positive.

BRAIN CHANGES

A healthy brain can and does change over time. It forms new connections to help us to learn new things throughout our lifetime. In depression, we see a lot of those connections lost over time.

Through brain imaging techniques such as MRI, scientists have noticed that specific brain regions shrink in depression. The memory region of the hippocampus and nearby areas that convey the meaning behind those memories (PFC and ACC) are smaller in depressed patients. They shrink because of a loss of grey matter (neurons and synapses), especially in areas of the brain responsible for our emotional thoughts and how we view not only the world, but ourselves. The emotional content of our daily experiences is a crucial aspect to maintaining our mental health and it likely has a big impact on our inner thoughts and feelings during depression.

Another area, called the *dentate gyrus* in the hippocampus, dramatically shrinks in untreated depressed patients compared with treated patients.[50] This brain region is part of the memory area too, and it helps the brain form new memories. It has received a lot of attention from scientists attempting to understand the link between depression and our ability to connect positive emotional content with new memories in the usual way.

STRESS – ONE OF THE BIGGEST ENEMIES OF THE BRAIN

How exactly does depression lead to changes in the brain? Scientists don't have all of the answers for that one, but what is known is that chronic stress is one reason why it could be happening. We know this because, amongst other things, smaller brain regions have been observed in the hippocampus and dentate gyrus of rodents who experience chronic stress.[51]

The body is very sensitive to stress, especially long-term, chronic stress. The HPA (hypothalamic–pituitary–adrenal) axis is the stress control centre of the brain and sends out hormones to help deal with it. Poor regulation of the HPA axis during depression leads to higher than normal levels of the stress hormone *cortisol*. This has been correlated with poor treatment responses and an increased chance of depression reoccurring. With this in mind, it would make sense for treatments to focus on the HPA axis as a way of trying to restore balance, but so far any attempts to modify it have not really worked, meaning scientists still need to understand a lot more about how it influences depression.

A recent study looked at a specific group of neurons within the hypothalamus (the *arcuate nucleus*), normally activated by food and hunger or emotional responses.[52] What the research team found was that unpredictable stress, like the unexpected death of a friend or family member, meant that these specific neurons became less active. They stopped working the way they should, and this may be one reason why isolated traumatic events can send someone into a downward spiral of depression. But the interesting thing is that these neurons could be tricked into working again, which reversed some depression-like symptoms in animals. Although it is difficult to replicate true depression in animal studies, the team think they have found the missing link they have been searching for. This subset of specific neurons that are turned off during depression and are active in people without it may just be crucial in how we deal with sudden stressful events. This is important because medications could eventually be created that would artificially dial these neurons up, reversing symptoms and the underlying neurobiology of depression.

Another important player in the stress game is brain-derived neurotrophic factor, or BDNF for short. It is a protein that keeps neurons alive and encourages them to grow, and it is crucial in helping the brain deal with stress. When BDNF levels are lower than normal, we are more vulnerable to the effects of stress on our health. What's more is that the levels of BDNF are reduced in the brain during depression and increased when antidepressants are taken, and closely align with a patient's symptoms. Because of observations like these, scientists believe BDNF may influence how the brain regions shrink during depression. We still need to understand why BDNF changes in certain people but sometimes, the changes result from the DNA that codes for it being slightly altered. This alteration means that each neuron's DNA blueprint is different, causing downstream problems that ultimately lead to the loss of grey matter and the shrinking of certain brain regions. This process has consistently been observed in the hippocampus, for example – an area important not only for memory function, but also for our emotional networks. The influence of the BDNF alteration is so great that merely having this change increases the chances of developing depression at some stage in our lives.

Although scientists think there may be a genetic component to depression, that is, DNA plays a role, because close family members have about a three times greater chance of developing depression, it is still unclear as to why some people suffer from it and others don't. Or why some people go through multiple episodes in their lifetime or find themselves resistant to many types of treatment. Genetic risks only leave a person having a greater susceptibility to depression, rather than a guarantee of depression, however – genes are not the entire story.

Early-life stress plays a big role in developing depression as an adult. It can cause changes to how our genes function, a field of study called epigenetics. For example, this stress can affect how BDNF works in our brain, alter neurons in the HPA axis, and one study looking at post-mortem brain tissue has even shown how child abuse can cause the long axons of neurons to lose some of their insulation (which helps them transmit signals better) in the ACC.[53]

It is not just the DNA we are born with, but how our body handles stress and trauma, that can have serious consequences to our mental health.

WHY IS THERE A LINK BETWEEN DEPRESSION AND HEART DISEASE?

It may be a little surprising to hear that chronic depression is linked to heart disease. As far as we know, there is no strong evidence to suggest that the changes occurring in the brain during depression directly cause heart disease. Similarly, scientists don't believe that the changes to the brain– gut axis directly lead to heart disease either, so what is going on?

It is suspected that there is an increased risk of developing heart disease the longer a person suffers from depression because of the additional effects depression has on lifestyle. Low mood and lack of motivation, over time, can lead to a more sedentary lifestyle and a drop in standards of self-care, particularly when it comes to diet and nutrition. Severe depression can leave a person with a low desire to start a new healthy routine, cook meals or even leave the house.

As we have seen already, changes in the brain can have a real effect, and contribute to lower levels of reward and motivation, and forward planning. Therefore, it has been suggested that the link between heart disease and depression results from an unhealthy lifestyle over many years, eventually contributing to health issues.

EXERCISE

The good news is that there are lots of very smart scientists and medical professionals out there who are determined to find new ways to help. Although neuroscientists have uncovered some mechanisms regarding how people develop depression, such as a neurotransmitter imbalance (*the monoamine hypothesis*), stress or even our DNA, the immense variability between patients suggests that there are a considerable amount of lifestyle effects that play some role in depression.

The so-called *lifestyle treatments* aimed at improving any additional factors, like diet, exercise, social or work stress and sleep, have been shown to be as effective in treating moderate depression as taking medication.[54] The idea here is that because a person may be more susceptible to a negative emotional state just because of the hardships of life, this may leave them more vulnerable to depression. Therefore, if we can remove some of those susceptibilities, it may reduce their chance of developing severe depression, offering at least some benefit to people.

Take exercise for example. It has been rated as the most beneficial lifestyle change towards improving the symptoms of depression. What's even more interesting is that exercise has been demonstrated to increase the size of the hippocampus, ACC and PFC in the brain.[55] As we discussed earlier, these areas are particularly important because their volume is reduced in depression, which may underpin some of the processes that cause symptoms. Depression slows the generation of new neurons, a process called *neurogenesis*, which our old favourite BDNF regulates. What is so exciting about the idea of exercise is that it has been shown to promote BDNF and actually increase neurogenesis in the brain.[56]

Other lifestyle treatments are designed to focus on different aspects that people may suffer with, and animal therapy is one example, aimed at improving positive emotions and boosting serotonin levels.[57] By interacting with pets or animals, both depression and anxiety levels can be significantly lowered. Although there are impressive early indications about its potential, it remains to be known how to best use this type of treatment. For example, which animals to use, for how long or how often and whether they should be used in combination with other strategies such as medications would be questions that need to be answered.

Naturally, using lifestyle treatments alone may not be sufficient for some people, especially those with more severe symptoms of depression, but the research is leading us to think that when used in combination with other treatments (the precise combination would depend on the individual) they may be able to offer some benefit.

WHAT HAPPENS IN THE BRAIN DURING MEDITATION – ARE THERE ANY REAL BENEFITS?

In recent years, mindfulness and meditation have become increasingly popular amongst those of us looking for a way to rebalance our inner thoughts against the backdrop of an ever more hectic work and life schedule. The potential benefits seem great – better sleep, reduced anxiety and improved focus – but do they really work?

There are countless books, courses and magazine articles that guide a person from novice to expert in no time at all, making big claims as they do it. Nevertheless, there is a danger of creating hype with all fashionable trends that science can't back up with any substantial evidence.

So, what does the science actually tell us then? Does meditation alter the brain in some way, either in the short term, or with lasting effects? Is it worth leaving the 9–5 and converting your house into a temple of meditation and peaceful contemplation?

There are many different types of meditation, each with their own unique benefits, so we will stick to mindfulness meditation for this question. Mindfulness is a process where you learn to pay attention to your thoughts and feelings in a very particular way, with more purpose and no judgement. In other words, it is a way to clear your mind just enough so that you can focus on what you are feeling physically, mentally or spiritually.

The entire basis for meditation is built on the idea that you can reset some of the neural networks within your brain that link the emotional areas to the more conscious centres – pretty much what you would think of as your inner thoughts. In neuroscience, this is called the default mode network (DMN).[a] Basically, it is what your brain is doing when you don't give it anything to do – when it is ticking over, waiting for the next thing to happen. You may think that if you are not really doing anything, like reading or talking, for example, your brain would have some downtime and be relaxing. Not so! At rest, your brain accounts for around 20% of all energy consumption in the body, meaning that the DMN is actually very important and can be highly active, particularly in mood disorders like depression. This network of our awareness and emotional responses is responsible for things like self-reflection, spontaneous thought and mind-wandering. Yes, there is an actual brain process for mind-wandering!

During meditation, exercises help reduce the activity of the DMN between some of the more influential regions of this network, like the amygdala. The amygdala appears a lot throughout our emotional processes. Once thought to be the fear centre and nothing more, we now view it as an important control region for our emotional responses. As meditation reduces the DMN activity, it has been reliably demonstrated to help with depression-related feelings, especially with self-reflection and recurring negative thoughts.[58] In fact, the

---

[a] Footnote: The DMN is a series of brain regions that are active when the brain is given no task, and quiet when the brain is busy doing something. You don't need to memorise all of the regions but the DMN includes the posterior cingulate cortex, lateral temporal cortex, medial PFC, parietal cortex, precuneus and hippocampus.

practice of mediation can be so positive that it can reduce depression relapse rates.[59]

The benefits for depression from the long-term practice of meditation may also be linked to an increase in grey matter (the neuron and its synapses) in the brain's frontal cortex. Our conscious thoughts are generated here, and by focusing on the inner thoughts while meditating it can help to increase brain cell density. Increasing the grey matter means more neurons and synapses, which may help to improve somebody's ability to self-reflect and recognise various emotional states. This is important because brain scans done during episodes of depression can often show a shrinkage in brain regions that have been linked with symptom severity (for a quick reminder, feel free to revisit the question on depression). In addition to all of this, meditation has also been shown to increase serotonin levels in the brain, which are a primary target of antidepressants. The very act of sitting and meditating may be enough to alter your brain in a genuine way.

There is also a substantial benefit for people who suffer with anxiety. An analysis which looked at nearly 50 studies for anxiety suggested that meditation could be used to successfully improve symptoms in as little as eight weeks.[60] There is also some evidence that it could be beneficial in post-traumatic stress disorder, ADHD and eating disorders, and it has been linked with better attention levels in day-to-day life, especially if you have practiced meditation for years.[61]

A cautionary tale though. Recent research is starting to suggest that there may also be negative and unpleasant experiences during meditation. When more than 1,200 regular meditators described their experience, over 25% stated that they occasionally had an unpleasant experience, often involving repetitive negative thinking during some of their meditation routines.[62] What is interesting, and yet to be explained, is that most of these people were trained at various meditation retreats, rather than teaching themselves at home.

Fear not though, because this upsetting meditation experience, although common, is largely related to the type of meditation, such as Vipassana style, which focuses intensely on insight into your own psyche. In other words, these distressing experiences arise from personal approaches to how we express and process our emotional experiences, and ruminating on them during meditation can sometimes lead to unpleasant reactions.

The reason that meditation can affect us so powerfully is because the DMN is very influential in our emotional regulation. Think about all of the times you have been sitting down and not doing much, and just how active your mind is. Learning to acknowledge these thoughts and regulate them into a more manageable process, as happens with meditation, is bound to impact many areas of your stressful daily life. Mostly, this is beneficial to people, but unfortunately, it may also be the reason for some of the unpleasant thoughts that some people experience.

If you want to give it a try for yourself, why not use music to help you? New and unfamiliar, repetitive and melodic music increases the emotional benefit from meditation – which can only be a good thing!

Do Men and Women Have Different Brains?

This sounds like a simple question to answer. Scan the brain, run some tests and voila, you have your answer! However, for every published article out there describing major differences between the sexes, there is an equal number of studies telling us that there are no differences, or at least, the differences are much smaller than people are led to believe.

The truth is that modern science has yet to offer a conclusive argument for either one, which tells us that although there may be individual differences within each study, there is no real difference between the brain of a man or woman – or at least none that you would notice in your everyday life.

The impact of our environment (in science terms, this is any change in the body that isn't caused by your DNA blueprint) on how we change and adapt has caused strong gender roles to be established. Women are often thought of as more emotional, empathetic and caring, whereas men are more geared towards logic and critical thinking. These biases creep into the scientific studies themselves, as we want to find the differences to support our views, which makes interpreting some of the science a little more difficult.

A team of researchers in the USA is one of several using brain imaging to look at the connectivity between the two sides of the brain (hemispheres) in men and women.[63] They did, in fact, observe differences between the sexes, detailing how male brains tended to be well connected within each individual hemisphere, and female brains were better connected between the two, a difference suggested to be linked with oestrogen levels. However, this study only looked at the brain during adolescence, a time when the brain undergoes a lot of development, and so may not explain the differences in adult brains accurately.

Along with studies demonstrating well-organised connectivity between the two brain hemispheres, which would result in messages being coordinated more efficiently throughout the entire brain, numerous studies suggest that there is much more grey matter in female brains.[64] Grey matter is where the neurons, glial cells and synapses are, as opposed to white matter, where the long myelin-coated axons of the neurons are. Interestingly, women tend to have a better outcome from brain injuries than men, and it is thought to be because of how oestrogen influences the glial cells in women. It has been known for a while that oestrogen can be protective in the brain, helping reduce inflammation, but it has also been observed to help create more glial cells, by up to 30%, aiding recovery from traumatic brain injuries.[65]

It has been suggested that the increased grey matter in women is centred around areas such as the medial PFC, OFC and posterior insula, whereas men tend to have more in the visual cortex, cerebellum and motor areas.[66] The more consistent view, on the other hand, is that when the results are properly adjusted for relative brain size and age, the differences are not as clearly defined. This is surprising considering a study by a team in Spain who declared that women outperformed men in fine-motor coordination, reading and writing ability, but testing characteristics like these depends heavily on factors that cannot be controlled for in a laboratory setting.[67] For example, the development of a person throughout their life, their interests, hobbies, learning and experience, will affect these characteristics.

Despite many structural differences being consistently observed, the underlying problem is that there is little functional difference. This means that although some structures may show observable differences in brain imaging, they don't really mean a whole lot – certainly nothing that would ever be noticed by someone.

The measurable differences are specific enough that Mireille Nieuwenhuis and colleagues described being able to tell apart the male and female brain only by the differences in brain structure.[68] In contrast to this, a study that looked at nearly 250,000 people found no differences between brains, and moreover that any small differences observed within the studies depended on the type of test done, giving different results each time.[69] This was especially the case when researchers tried to test these differences with cognitive tasks. In other words, if you give a book about Shakespeare to a group of females, and another about Harry Potter to males, you will see differences in how they each describe and relate to the book. Frankly, that doesn't really mean the brains are different in each group. Some will simply like Harry Potter more than Shakespeare.

Many differences between the two sexes appear throughout the scientific literature as a result of different brain sizes. On average, men have 11% larger brain size, which some scientists suggest results in a greater number of neurons and an increased intelligence or IQ.[70] But – and it is a big but – if the data are adjusted for the brain's relative size to the body, these differences disappear. When we look at it in a more forensic way, there is absolutely no difference in IQ between brains, regardless of sex. This has been consistently proven.[71]

Men and women are different though, so what about the hormones? Clearly, there are differences in hormones between the sexes. Oestrogen and progesterone are predominantly seen in females, with testosterone underlying many developmental effects in males (although both males and females have all of these – yes, men have oestrogen). Hormonal changes in times of development may account for differences, particularly in younger study participants. But differences are also caused by lifestyle effects and cause the body and brain to change over time (called *epigenetic* changes). This is important because it is one reason why we don't see any reliable functional differences between sexes: the brain adapts and rewires itself to accomplish a task to get the same results as another brain. If anything, it describes how the plasticity of the brain can be programmed in one of many ways to wire the brain to achieve the same result.

The brains may look different, but they compensate for it and work just as well as each other. Experimental research can never replicate the individual differences in human beings, and the general consensus in the research is that, although there may be subtle differences in the brains of men and women, there is also much overlap and individual variation, resulting in no difference between the two sexes.

What is our consciousness?

It may seem obvious to explain to someone that you are conscious. I mean, you talk, you think, you laugh and smile, you read neuroscience books, so you are conscious – right?

Typically, we would define consciousness as an awareness of the world around us and our personal experience within it. Although we have an intrinsic awareness that we are conscious, and can consciously experience the world, when we come to define what that means scientifically, things get a lot more tricky.

For example, if we as humans are conscious, then how conscious are animals? Is it the same as our level of consciousness? What about trees? What about the chair you are sitting on? OK, now what about a computer that thinks and talks like we do? Where do we draw the line and how do we define consciousness in a way that befits a neuroscience book?

One of the reasons it is so difficult for scientists to prove or define consciousness is the remarkably high number of interactions in the brain. They each influence their own set of interactions, together with the extremely subjective definitions of an experience, making it a very complex thing to study. What neuroscientists need are markers of consciousness. Things that the brain, or body, do that tell us 'Yes, this is it, we are conscious and living the high life right now.'

To measure consciousness uniformly, there needs to be a way to link what we experience during the day to the neural mechanisms inside the brain. We need to be able to *see* it. This requires assessing all of the inputs the brain receives from the world around us: things like auditory, visual and verbal inputs, along with any movement that the body makes. A combination of all of these would give a perception of one's own awareness and conscious experience. To put it another way, scientists can measure specific parts of the brain all at once to see how it is using all of that information, and if we are truly aware of it. This works well when you think about being awake compared with sleeping, or being in a coma or otherwise unconscious. Our conscious experience changes because when we are sleeping, we are clearly not aware of these inputs, at least not to the extent that we would be during wakefulness.

To make things more complicated, scientists can't simply use an EEG device to measure brain waves and activity, because consciousness is a lot more specific and subtle than that. The measurements from EEG recordings don't align with consciousness as well as you might think. This has led scientists to believe that how we experience consciousness results from smaller, specific regions in the brain communicating with one another, rather than a more global effect.

What neuroscientists *can* do, is look at brain activity when a person is awake and conscious, compared with when they are not, such as during sleep or being under anaesthesia. Functional MRI scans are perfectly capable of distinguishing these changes in activity patterns as a person regains consciousness after anaesthesia.[72] Judging by data like this, one hypothesis about consciousness states that it is merely our brain's way of interpreting information from our senses.

There is so much information all coming in at the same time, that over the course of evolution the brain has learned to simultaneously compute this information into what we perceive as consciousness. It is nothing more than our brain's output of all the input. As a way to help us thrive in our environment, the brain creates an avatar, or an out-of-body experience, to summarise all this information. By doing this, we can think in a more complex way, imagining ourselves in someone else's shoes, looking back at ourselves, and we have this avatar or perspective in our mind as our inner thoughts.

Imagine a computer. It is built with hardware – computer chips, wires and the rest of it. Collectively, it runs an operating system, such as Windows, which in turn runs a program you want, like a word processor. Consciousness may be very similar: our brain's neurons send and receive signals that, collectively, form complex operating systems, which culminate in a program, or a conscious experience of the world around us. It may be nothing more than sensory inputs, on a grand scale.

What about our subconscious? An experiment by Libet and colleagues showed something exciting. They asked people to make simple movements while their brain activity was recorded.[73] What it showed was that the brain decides to move approximately 0.5 seconds before we are ever aware of it. Considering neurons send signals in the thousandths of a second, half a second is a very long time in the brain (0.5 seconds is 500 thousandths). This result is rather a controversial one. Some scientists believe that the methods used to test this timing were deeply flawed and provided a result that was neither accurate nor useful. More recent studies have accepted the result, and even put the time delay at nearly 1.5 seconds, three times longer than originally thought.[74]

So, what is going on in this half a second? It suggests that there is a clear and defined difference between subconscious and conscious awareness and that we are only able to perceive a glimpse of this process. It could very well be that our subconscious, which on many occasions heavily influences our conscious thoughts, is the real driver of our conscious experience, and our inner thoughts are just the brain's way of explaining some of that detail to us. More philosophically, our consciousness could essentially be an autopilot for our subconscious behaviours, for which we are not ever truly able to experience a full version of reality.

In this regard, less-developed brains, such as those in animals, will also experience consciousness, although probably not in the same way we do. We know that animals experience a range of emotions, have some form of 'personality', and even demonstrate complex emotional responses like empathy. With a higher level of consciousness comes more self-awareness. Dolphins, along with a select few animals like elephants and chimpanzees, are some of the only mammals to recognise themselves in the reflection of a mirror, rather than assuming it is another animal in close proximity. This in itself raises more questions about the level of consciousness that animals are aware of, and how they understand the world.

Our current understanding of our own consciousness (still very much lacking) would hypothesise that the consciousness of animals would be much more basic, with things like subconscious thoughts and more complicated levels of perception mostly absent. Fundamental thoughts regarding food, shelter and predators may come as instinctual behaviours rather than as how humans would experience them, such as complex thoughts, internal dialogues and well-thought-out decisions – although this will vary from species to species. In reality though, we may never really know.

If consciousness really is just a collection of neuronal inputs then what inputs are necessary? We know that the frontoparietal lobes are essential for our being awake and conscious of our experiences, but we don't know to what extent. It may be that they are more important in interpreting our consciousness experience for our inner thoughts and behaviours but may not be essential themselves in creating consciousness. Even if we start to understand some of the brain regions involved in consciousness, we need another level of understanding. What type of neurons are essential, what combination of signalling needs to occur and what signalling pattern causes our experiences are all questions that science has yet to answer.

Indeed, it has been proposed that consciousness may be all around us at any given moment, and we simply experience it as we live our lives. It doesn't exist in our thoughts, and it certainly isn't created by our mere presence, but rather we feel its ebb and flow, as if we are swimming in an ocean of consciousness that we can feel and experience, just as we would feel the water, but it is not really ours to explain or take ownership of.

If we think back to the neurobiology of consciousness, which scientists believe is the culmination of our neural networks, then we should be able to alter our experience of consciousness at will, right? Anyone who has taken psychedelic drugs will probably explain that very well. Sleep, drugs and anaesthesia all change our perception of reality, but none more so than the drug *dextromethorphan*. This results in side effects that cause time distortion, dissociation from your own experiences, hallucinations, euphoria and many other psychological effects. Understanding how compounds like dextromethorphan produce their effects may explain some of the reasons we experience the world the way we do. For example, we know that the drug acts to increase serotonin in the brain, and although it is not completely understood, it somehow blocks glutamate receptors, which are potent stimulators of neurons. This understanding would fit nicely with the neurobiology of consciousness, which states that it is simply a combination of neural activities, likely utilising serotonin and glutamate.

On a last note, some people refer to our consciousness as our soul – the thing which is required to experience life, and without it, we die. Some believe that the soul will return to an afterlife at the time of death, yet people who express an alternative viewpoint say that, in fact, nothing happens at this moment. We simply cease to exist and do not continue to experience any form of consciousness. Who really knows which option is correct, but what really fascinates me, is that when asked to describe what that would be like, experiencing nothingness, people almost always say, 'Well, what was it like before you were born?' This is bizarre! Although I clearly have no idea what happens and prefer not to think about it, it always strikes me as strange that people stick memory and consciousness together and assume that consciousness cannot exist without memory. It could be that before birth, there is a multitude of experiences that we are consciously aware of, but we simply have no memory of them. If we think back to the memory question, memory formation requires a brain, and for the most part, neuronal connections to the hippocampus. We know that people with severe injuries resulting in very limited memory abilities are still conscious and experiencing life.

Take one example. If you are playing sports and suffer a head injury that results in amnesia, you may never recall the game, or the entire day in which you played. But you certainly had feelings, emotions and a general experience, even if you don't remember it. And I am reasonably sure that a three-week-old child is conscious, regardless of the fact that we can never recall being a three-week-old baby. In this regard, not remembering doesn't discount the conscious experience.

Consciousness is very subjective and who is to say what it really is? Science is yet to provide a conclusive answer, so perhaps we may never fully understand it.

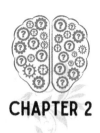

CHAPTER 2

THE X-FILES OF NEUROSCIENCE

INTRODUCTION

Hopefully, after reading the first part of this book, you have gained a greater appreciation for how our brain works, and quite frankly, just how little we truly understand about the body's sophisticated computer. Together, we have explored some of the beauty behind the intricate and marvellous processes our brain goes through each day. But what happens when the brain doesn't work quite as we expect?

As neuroscientists, we are able to observe and record the activity of the brain, and yet we do not fully appreciate why this activity occurs in the first place, and so the challenge of a neuroscientist is not only to observe these curiosities but to ask why. Why do some people remember everything that has ever happened to them and others do not? Why do some of us have a sudden urge to jump off a tall building for apparently no reason?

This next chapter explores some of the most exciting and curious phenomena in the brain and the consequences we may experience as a result of them. By studying the brain when it isn't working the way it should, we can learn a great deal and start to unravel a tiny piece of the puzzle, one step at a time. Some of the phenomena below are perfect examples of instances when, despite how impressive our brain can be, it can be easily confused, tricked or influenced. Enjoy!

THE BAADER-MEINHOF PHENOMENON

The Baader–Meinhof phenomenon (pronounced bar-der mine-hof), also called the frequency illusion, is one I am sure most of you have experienced at some point already. The term is linked to an incident in 1994 when a man noted that upon hearing the name Baader–Meinhof (actually the name of a 1970s terrorist group from Germany),[a] he then overheard it in multiple conversations over the next 24 hours. After years of study into this phenomena, in 2006, Arnold Zwicky, a Stanford linguistics professor, called it the Baader–Meinhof phenomenon.

This phenomenon occurs when your awareness of something specific increases for a short period of time. It often happens when you have recently learned a new word, and you notice everyone using it in conversation, or that it frequently appears on signs or websites or in newspapers. Perhaps you have just bought a new car, and now you see the same model all over the roads. Of course, it could also be that people saw just how great you look driving the car and collectively decided to try and be more like you.

There is a relatively simple explanation for this phenomenon, and it relates to how much attention the brain devotes to everything around us. There is an extraordinary number of stimuli in everyday life, from sounds, smells and colour, each with their own subtle details. Take a person, for example. You could systematically look them up and down and notice everything about their appearance – jewellery, posture, clothing – or the perfume they are wearing. For the brain, this is simply too much information to process at one time, in any

---

[a] A reference to the Baader–Meinhof gang, or Red Army Faction, also appears in a 2018 remake of *Suspiria*, by Luca Guadagnino.

great detail. Therefore, it becomes selective and chooses to focus on only one major detail at any given time. The attention span of the brain can be surprisingly short, and so it gets excited by finding something new. The Baader–Meinhof phenomenon works because as the brain learns new things it devotes more attention to the new item you have noticed, as if to say, 'Hey look, here it is again, it must be important.' It is more consciously aware of the new item and will prioritise it over other things – meaning that if you hear about it in conversation, or read about it somewhere else, your brain will easily notice, and you feel as if it is everywhere you look.

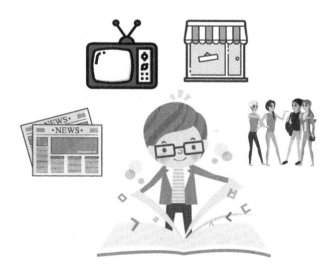

Have you ever noticed this phenomenon? You learn a new word, and suddenly it is everywhere!

CONGENITAL INSENSITIVITY TO PAIN

Nobody likes stubbing their toe in the middle of the night, but that feeling of pain is actually crucial in teaching us that we shouldn't do it again. This seems obvious, but there is a considerable amount of programming that took millions of years of evolution to develop into the precise pain system we have today. The pain exists as a way for your brain to alert you to any dangers that may threaten your survival. Therefore, because we don't like pain, we tend to stay away from dangerous things. At least most of us do.

Some people don't feel any pain at all, regardless of what they do. Congenital insensitivity to pain (CIP) occurs when neurons that send pain messages to the brain fail to correctly detect a painful stimulus and convert it to a signal. These neurons are called nociceptors, and the signals they send are called action potentials.

The endings of our nociceptors have many receptors and 'channels'. These channels open or remain closed, and by doing so, they alter the amount of positive or negative ions passing through the neuron's membrane, so we have cleverly called them ion channels.[a] Since the action potential is an electrical signal, these neurons rely heavily on ion channels to synchronise the voltage changes along the neuron, which is basically a long electrical cable anyway. A gene mutation[b] affecting one of the ion channels sensitive for sodium results

[a] Amongst other things, ion channels are responsible for some of the electrical properties of a neuron, such as building up the voltage needed to fire off an action potential.

[b] The *SCN9A* gene mutation leads to alterations in the alpha subunit of the Nav1.7 ion channel, which is important in action potential generation. A mutation to this gene can lead to alterations in nociceptor function, including a loss of pain sensitivity or hypersensitivity to pain.

in a nociceptor that can't cause a significant enough change in the voltage to trigger an action potential, and so the brain doesn't get the pain message. It's like putting your friend in a big catapult with an important letter to send, and only by hand. They sit in the catapult and wait for you to draw them back with enough elasticity to fling them forward for miles, flying majestically through the air. To create enough force, you need many people to draw the catapult backwards, just like the neuron needs a lot of ion channels. Without enough, even if the message of pain (or the letter) is written, it isn't even going to launch. It will just sit there in a strange mediaeval catapult wondering why the author didn't write an analogy with a more comfortable seat.

With CIP, even if you were to cut yourself or burn your hand, as far as the nociceptor is concerned, it simply carries on life as usual. Although CIP was first reported in 1932, the mutation is so rare that it has only recently been studied in detail. Neuroscientists are looking at these voltage-gated sodium channels to develop pain medication based on the principles of CIP.

What is really interesting about how our body feels pain, is that it only exists because of signals coming from outside the brain, and that's why injuring the brain itself would not be painful. Neurosurgeons can slice and dissect your brain without you feeling any discomfort, provided local anaesthesia helps with the initial surgical incision to your head. As the brain relies on these messages coming from your body to produce pain, it seemingly never occurred to it to develop a detection method for itself. Think of it a little bit like receiving a letter from a family member in another city. The postman delivers it to your house, and you read it, and decide how to respond. However, in order to receive a letter, you need an external family member to post it to you. It wouldn't make much sense to mail a letter to yourself, wait for it to arrive, and reply to yourself with another letter, so the brain doesn't send pain signals to itself.

Although living without pain may sound like a sort of superpower and one which many of us have considered at a moment of agony, I'm sure, it is anything but a superpower. Life for a person living with this condition is complicated. As children, they often find themselves with minor or even significant injuries and little awareness of their consequences. Daily checks and a more structured lifestyle are needed to avoid considerable harm from unknown injuries.

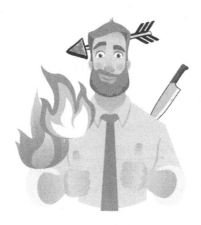

Just think of all the things that would no longer hurt. Just in case they do hurt, please don't try this at home.

CAPGRAS SYNDROME

This entry into the X-Files of neuroscience is fascinating, albeit a little heartbreaking. Capgras syndrome is a specific situation where familiar people seem like strangers. Your mother may look like herself, sound the same and even have the same memories as her, and yet you do not recognise her as your mother, only a lookalike or imposter. This delusion may also be transferred to objects such as your house, whereby you believe you are viewing another home, even though you realise it is very similar to your own. Capgras syndrome is often a symptom of a psychiatric disorder or dementia, but can also be caused by brain injury, infection or drug abuse.

Named after the French psychiatrist Joseph Capgras, who first described this phenomenon in 1923, it would have been an odd and unusual symptom to rationalise, and even a century later, the precise reasons remain a mystery. In 1991, M. David Enoch and William (Bill) Trethowan[1] attempted to solve this mystery by seeing it not as a neurological abnormality, but as a psychological dispute with your own inner love-hate conflict, directing hate towards the imposter but retaining a love for the original person.

This may help to explain the relationship with familiar people, but it fails to explain why this delusion spreads to objects and locations such as a person's house. From a neuroscience point of view, it is thought to involve the visual and memory parts of our brains, and how they are connected to our emotional areas throughout the limbic system. This would explain why the brain can recognise a familiar person yet is unable to couple it with the correct emotional context, resulting in your mother feeling like a woman you may know but have no emotional connection with.

This seems sensible when we consider the following case study, where a man developed Capgras syndrome after a car accident had left him with a traumatic brain injury.[2] After apparently recovering well he was able to identify his parents but only as imposters who looked and acted like them. Rather interestingly, this was not the case if they were talking over the phone, when he would readily accept that they were his parents. Scientists concluded that when the visual cortex in the brain wasn't needed, such as when speaking on the telephone and not speaking with his parents in person, the memories and emotional context remained coupled, meaning he could freely engage with his parents without any delusional distractions. This adds to the weight of evidence suggesting that Capgras syndrome results from a disconnection between the visual and emotional regions in the brain.

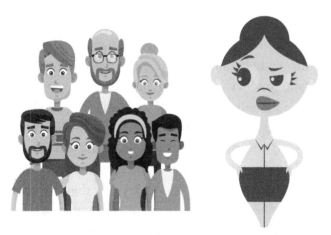

Can you imagine how strange it would feel to see someone you know, yet still do not recognise?

Another case study from a 77-year-old woman explains even more of this phenomenon. She was found by her son talking to a person in the mirror. Being deaf, she was using sign language, and when asked about this other woman in the mirror, she told her son that although she looked similar to herself and even had a similar life story, she could not possibly be the same person. She knew this because of the poor use of sign language from the other woman. She could identify other reflections in the mirror as simply reflections, but her own would appear to her as a new person. What neuroscience tells us is that the part of our brain responsible for facial recognition is predominantly in the right hemisphere. When scientists studied her brain, it became apparent that there was a noticeable reduction in the size of the temporoparietal region on the right side of the brain, an area involved in cognition, memory and language, which may help to explain some of these occurrences. Although we understand the brain at a much deeper level than in 1923, Capgras syndrome is not yet fully understood, but cases such as these may help neuroscientists to discover more.

A STRANGE FACE IN THE MIRROR

Speaking of reflections in the mirror, even with a healthy brain, it is possible for your own reflection to seem like it is another person looking back at you. They don't necessarily have to be alive, or even a human. In 2010 an Italian psychologist named Giovanni Caputo performed an experiment[3] with 50 people who, one by one, were sat in front of a mirror under dim lighting and asked to stare at their own reflection. Each person reported seeing their face deformed, seeing the faces of their parents (some of whom were not alive any more) or even seeing animal faces. What is more remarkable is that you do not even need a mirror. Five years later, the experiment was repeated,[4] this time with test subjects looking into the eyes of someone else sitting opposite them. Each person experienced the same strange hallucinations lasting 7 seconds, experiencing a couple of hallucinations every minute. If you are feeling brave, you may want to try this experiment yourself.

Initially, there was a lot of debate as to why this occurs. It has been suggested that these temporary hallucinations are part of our subconscious being projected onto another person's body. However, a much more likely explanation is that when we stare at an unchanging face for an extended time, the visual neurons in our brain get used to it and start to decrease their activity, believing it to be less important to us, and so we observe facial features that begin to blur and disappear. Furthermore, facial mimicry and contagion are considered to be important in this phenomenon. These are instances where we change our facial expressions or actions to mimic social behaviours from others, and so we may change the image we see into what our brain thinks would be appropriate.

As humans, we are extremely sensitive to reading facial expressions and will often unconsciously alter our own to appear more acceptable to others. It is because of this that the brain is always working, trying to understand our environment. Without enough of a stimulus (staring at an unchanging face is boring to the brain) it starts to fill in the gaps, leading to bizarre distortions coming out of prominent features on the face. The low lighting conditions probably add a little to the effect by causing minor sensory deprivation, which confuses our brain even more.

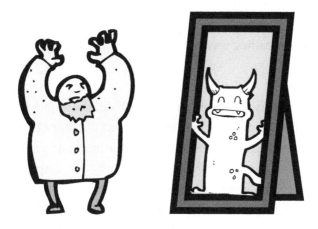

Do you feel brave enough to give this a try? See if you can replicate the findings from previous studies.

WAS IT MY FACE OR YOURS?

This seems like the perfect time to talk about faces. Specifically, why some people just can't seem to remember them, a term scientists call prosopagnosia or face blindness. A person with prosopagnosia cannot recognise familiar faces easily, and often can't distinguish between unknown faces like those of strangers. Prosopagnosia leads to difficulty in recalling visual memories not exclusively with faces but also with identifying landmarks or objects, which can make tasks like navigation particularly difficult. In the most severe cases, people may also have difficulty in recognising themselves. There remains a lot that is unclear about what happens in the brain during prosopagnosia, but it is thought that there is a connectivity problem between our visual areas and the memory centres in our brain. We know this because a person with prosopagnosia who recognises a familiar face can have difficulty recalling any details about the person if they leave the room.

Scientists believe there is a genetic component to prosopagnosia, with approximately 2% of the population born with some form of it. If you are born with it, there is evidence that it develops as a result of a defect in a part of the brain called the fusiform gyrus.[a] This area is implicated in recognising human faces in great detail and evolved to help us to identify the faces of our family and other members of our community. As such, it appears to be an area that is essentially preprogrammed with information, and developmental issues in the fusiform gyrus will lead to difficulties like prosopagnosia later on in life.

[a] Facial processing in the brain relies on the fusiform gyrus, occipital cortex and superior temporal sulcus to identify a person's face with exceptional specificity.

However, people are not only born with prosopagnosia but can acquire it throughout their lives, usually from a brain injury, stroke or a degenerative disease. Recent brain scans of a 65-year-old man who had noticed his prosopagnosia getting worse revealed shocking changes in the brain. The areas of the brain that process facial recognition and memories were shrinking, resulting in more severe face blindness[5] (the fusiform gyrus and the right side of the temporal lobe). These changes seemed to occur mostly in the right side of the brain, which contributes a lot to our visual processing.

Currently, there is no cure for prosopagnosia but rather a focus on practising compensatory skills such as memorising a person's clothing, or prominent characteristics about their appearance, which can lead to substantial improvements.

If any of this sounds familiar, there are several tests such as the Benton Facial Recognition Test (BFRT) or Cambridge Face Memory Test (CFMT). These tests rely on looking at a number of faces and pairing them with an identical one, or a face that you saw only moments ago.

It happens to all of us at some point. You just can't seem to remember who they are. Eventually, it goes on too long and it is too awkward to ask.

A WISE OLD BRAIN

A fun fact about your brain is that for the most part, the brain cells you are born with will continue to develop and grow as you learn, and actually stay with you for your entire life. The exact same ones! So, if you live to be 80, you will have 80-year-old brains, and if we can live that long, even 100 or 200 years old. Seems fairly old right? OK, now try 2,000 years old!

Picture the scene in the year 79 A.D. when a young man around 20 years of age (let's call him Aurelius) is feeling tired after a long day serving as guardian of the college of Herculaneum, an ancient city close to Naples, Italy. So, Aurelius decides to take a short nap in his bed. Then suddenly 20 kilometres away, Mount Vesuvius erupts, spewing out hot volcanic ash at 500°C, rapidly burying everything in 20 metres of ash, including our dear sleepy friend Aurelius.

Fast forward to the 1960s and Aurelius was found lying on a wooden bed under a pile of ash. By this time, the remains were not particularly recognisable, unlike some other victims we can see clearly today, but what was so exceptional is that Aurelius' preserved brain tissue was also discovered. The extreme heat and then rapid cooling typical of the volcanic ash from Mount Vesuvius meant that the brain cells were turned into a glassy material, almost freezing the cells intact. The brain cells kept structural features only found in the central nervous system, which helped to identify them as brain matter. A more recent study[6] even looked at his brain material under an extremely powerful electron microscope using new technology that allowed scientists to visualise the brain cells. The research team confirmed that they were studying the neurons from a spinal cord and brain by using X-ray spectroscopy[a] to identify organic material. The study was a great advert for this new way of researching ancient cellular material. This research will open a new line of biogeoarcheological investigations, and the team hope to use this method to search other sites around the world to uncover previously unknown areas of ancient burial grounds.

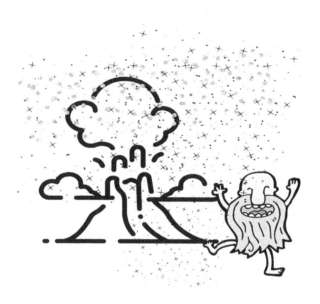

Although it is highly unlikely there were bearded old men dancing under the volcano as it erupted. We will never really know.

[a] X-ray spectroscopy measures X-rays in order to understand the different chemical properties of something. It helps to create a better idea of what it is that you're looking at.

PHINEAS GAGE

As neuroscientists, we can learn a lot from people in everyday life. It's not just laboratories and microscopes. This often means examining someone who has had a severe brain injury but who is alive and otherwise well. One of the most famous examples of this in neuroscience comes from a man named Phineas Gage. A 25-year-old construction worker who in 1848 was working on the construction of a new railroad when he accidentally set off an explosion that launched an iron bar into his skull and brain. The force of the blast was so great, the bar exited his head and landed on the other side of the track. To the amazement of everyone around him, he survived. Not long after his accident, Phineas Gage was able to talk, and with a little help, walk around. He recovered very well and didn't appear to show any early signs of a lowered intelligence, compromised speech or physical paralysis.

Despite his impressive recovery, people eventually started to notice changes in his personality. He became unreliable in his job, acting inappropriately in social situations and started frequently cursing, ultimately losing his job and dying only a few years later from a seizure. Gage went from being a polite, responsible and well-mannered man to someone entirely different; however, the true changes may never be known as much of his later story has been dramatised.

We now know that Gage suffered substantial damage to an area of the brain called the prefrontal cortex (PFC)[a] – an area that is important in decision-making, emotional processing and forming long-term memories. The reason that most of his mental faculties remained intact was because a smaller area

[a] Damage specifically to the medial PFC and left orbital PFC.

of the PFC (the dorsolateral PFC) was miraculously undamaged, and it is this area that is involved in many of the higher cognitive functions (things like goal-setting and problem-solving). The case of Phineas Gage was so intriguing to the field of neuroscience that his body was later exhumed so that his skull could be reconstructed using 3D computer technology, allowing us to understand the extent of his injuries.

The story of Phineas Gage is an unfortunate tale of a man who survived an injury yet suffered in life, and a reminder of how curious but tragic the study of neuroscience can be.

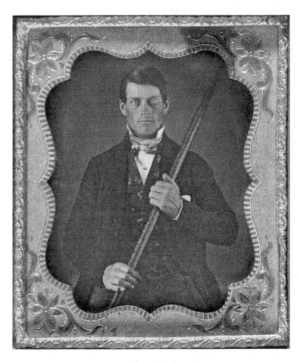

A shocking ordeal and an amazing story that deserves its place in neuroscience history.

HIGH PLACES PHENOMENON

Have you ever been standing at the top of a tall building or cliff edge and had a sudden but brief urge to jump? You have no real thought of actually doing it, and you are not depressed, suicidal or otherwise distressed, but that urge appears, nonetheless. As it turns out, neuroscience has a name for such an occurrence – the *high places phenomenon*, sometimes termed the *call to the void* – and it is actually very normal and common. There are also reports of impulses to jump in front of a train, stick a hand in a fire or turn a steering wheel into traffic. Thankfully, the person generally doesn't follow through, and although most accounts of this phenomenon are anecdotal, there is one team of scientists in Florida, USA, who decided to take another look.[7]

The research team asked 431 students about such episodes in their personal lives, and a surprising 55% acknowledged that they have experienced them at some stage in their lives. As neuroscientists, we are yet to comprehend why these thoughts occur, but evidence from this study highlighted increased levels of anxiety correlating with an increased frequency of these intrusive thoughts.[a] Anxiety, not uncommon amongst students, may have resulted in a higher frequency compared with the general public. Just why anxiety would influence this behaviour is yet to be studied.

Science has, however, revealed to us that the high place phenomenon is possibly the result of a split-second delay between two opposing brain signals. One signal is based on our survival instinct that notices danger and tells us that we

---

[a] Be aware that if these thoughts occur regularly and last longer than a brief moment it may be a sign of something more serious and you should consult a medical professional.

should avoid it, such as falling from a great height or a train hitting us in the face. Another signal coming from our more logical brain tells us that we are relatively safe where we are, and there is no real threat to our survival. The resulting signals are interpreted by our brain – now somewhat confused – for it to relay this rather bizarre message and we experience the high places phenomenon. So, if you ever have a sudden impulse to jump off the top of Mount Everest, just remember that it is normal, but please don't do it anyway.

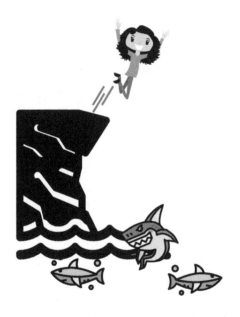

As much as you might want to sometimes, please don't jump from high places, especially if there are sharks below.

SENSING MAGNETIC FIELDS

It is well established that birds can sense the Earth's magnetic field and use this, along with landmarks, to navigate during flight. They are able to do this due to magnetic particles very close to nerve endings in their head, which translate sensory information about touch, temperature and pain, meaning that birds essentially 'feel' the magnetic field. The retinas of their eyes contain something called *cryptochrome*, a small protein that acts differently depending on the strength of the magnetic field. What is interesting is that scientists have discovered that humans have this cryptochrome too. Scientists at Caltech observed how the EEG (an electroencephalogram, which measures brain waves) of people changes when exposed to different magnetic fields.[8] This is harmless, and naturally occurs throughout our everyday lives, but this study was the first to report that humans may be able to sense this magnetic information and utilise it for themselves. Based on this research, some scientists have suggested that this may have helped our human ancestors to navigate between the North and South.

Conversely, many scientists are unconvinced and feel there may be no functional benefit to the low levels of cryptochrome, and that merely observing its presence doesn't translate to an effect. It is perhaps more reasonable to suggest that if there ever was a navigational benefit, it would have been lost over the course of our evolutionary history, and today's navigation relies on the logic, spatial awareness and memory centres of our brain.

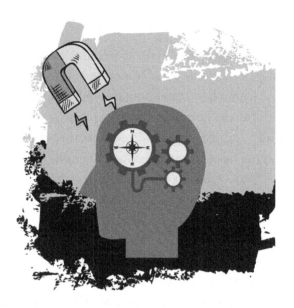

What do you think about this one? Can you navigate effortlessly? Maybe this is the reason why.

As of yet, there are no recorded cases of humans able to sense magnetic fields, which would be like having a sixth sense – allowing you to walk in the right direction without the need of a compass – but it is an interesting thought, nonetheless.

BLINDSIGHT

At the back of the brain we have the occipital lobe. This region receives images from our eyes and optic nerves and decides what we are seeing before sending that information to other parts of our brain to determine how to react. So, if we see an adorable fluffy dog, the light reflected from that dog travels to our retina at the back of our eye, along the optic nerve and to the occipital lobe, where it is processed by the primary and secondary visual cortices. Other areas (frontal cortex and limbic system) then interpret the meaning and decide what the emotional response should be, resulting in a very excited 'Aww, a cute puppy – I like this, I feel happy!'

However, damage to the occipital lobe, for example, through trauma, a brain tumour or a stroke, can result in the images of the cute puppy arriving at the visual cortex but not being processed or transmitted to other areas of our brain, and hence, we become blind. This is a little different to instances where the eyes or optic nerve don't function. This additional blindness is termed *cortical blindness* – essentially, blindness in the brain. You may be asking why this chapter is talking about cute puppies and blindness. Well, because in some people with cortical blindness, even though they can't see particular objects, their subconscious brain still perceives them. This means a person can interact with something even if they don't actually see it. Let's use another example. Say you want to walk across the room to the doorway, but there is a chair in your path. Under normal circumstances, you would see the chair and walk around it. A person with *blindsight* would also walk across the room and avoid the chair, yet they would not actively see that there is a chair in the room. They simply avoid it but do not fully understand why.

This strange phenomenon was first documented in the 1974 research by Lawrence Weiskrantz and has since been recorded in all manner of situations.[9] A person may catch a ball in mid-air without ever seeing it, for example, but perhaps the most interesting study shows how it is possible to identify facial emotions and even mirror those same emotions in your own face, without ever being consciously aware of seeing any facial expressions.

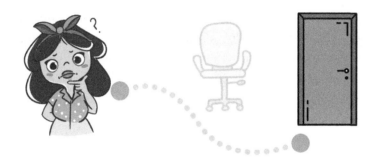

The brain is a really strange, but fascinating place that we may never fully comprehend.

Blindsight has been rigorously tested in many experimental settings, and as such, neuroscientists think they have an explanation. Firstly, the fact that some people with cortical blindness experience the phenomenon of blindsight may be because the *superior colliculus* – an area of the brain important in visual orientation – is preserved.[10] Although we don't yet fully appreciate the full function of the superior colliculus, we do know that this area receives information about what we see and converts it into signals that initiate an appropriate movement. To help explain this, imagine sitting down and watching a racing car drive past. Our eyes and head would instinctively follow the car as we track its movements. This is the responsibility of the superior colliculus, to instinctively monitor the environment and decide how to move our body.

The current hypothesis for blindsight states that as the brain senses damage to the occipital lobe, it starts to rewire itself to bypass the primary visual cortex, and with the help of the superior colliculus send the information through an area called the *lateral geniculate nucleus* in the centre of the brain. The person may never entirely regain normal vision, but they may still be capable of living a normal life. Some neuroscientists suggest that this is a process by which the brain reverts back to a more basic form of vision, and one that is seen in animals who naturally lack the advanced visual areas of a human brain.

PERFECT MEMORY

There is no such thing as a perfect memory, but as far as neuroscience teaches us, we never forget anything. Although in reality, most memories cannot be retrieved by us at a conscious level, and so you may think that they are lost forever. However, this forgetfulness is simply a mechanism that our brain utilises so we can easily remember the important things and not get distracted by the countless other memories we store. Some people do not appear to have that ability and instead live with a nearly perfect memory recall of their entire lives.

This is called *hyperthymesia*, and it gives people the ability to have a near-perfect autobiographical memory about their lives. To accurately recall every major news event, day by day, from previous years, or recall what day of the week it was on a random date from the past, even describing the menu from a restaurant they visited on that date. An account of the life of Jill Price, the first person to be identified as having this enhanced memory, recently described how, at the age of only eight, her brain suddenly changed.[11] From then, she could never seem to forget any detail from her life. This means she can remember every day from 1980 onwards, and although it is not quite a perfect memory, she can remember what she was doing, who she was with and where she was.

Scientists think that hyperthymesia may be similar to instances of acquired savant syndrome in which we see people develop extraordinary mental abilities in arithmetic and factual memory. Taking a closer look, brain scans have revealed differences in the brains of people with hyperthymesia compared with those with standard memory.[12] These include a larger *parahippocampal gyrus* (an area surrounding the memory region), which is associated with autobiographical memories and spatial awareness (where we are). Although we can identify these changes, they do not fully explain the difference in memory capabilities, meaning that it is more likely to be explained by how the brain stores its memories, rather than the size of specific areas.

This connectivity has recently been demonstrated between the temporal lobe (memory), parietal lobe (things like touch and taste) and the prefrontal cortex (analytical thought). These areas are important for memory and impressive analytical feats. In short, the brain does store these memories differently in the brain of someone like Jill Price, but they have better memories due to how easily they can be accessed. It is like your mind has a direct phone line to the memory centre, rather than going through layers of poorly organised filing cabinets of information.

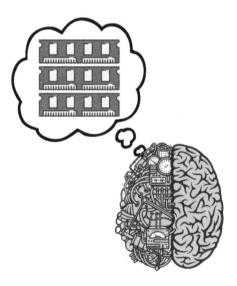

Would it be a good thing to always remember, or would it be bad? I think I would prefer to stick to my regular memory for now.

Neuroscientists are also able to observe differences in responses when asking people with hyperthymesia to describe themselves. People with hyperthymesia often have a more extraordinary imagination and absorption characteristics (the ability to be completely focused and attentive to the sensations of an activity). They often describe being more sensitive to sound, smell and visual stimuli, and the level of detail acquired through this sensitivity may help to make daily events much more memorable. In addition, it is not uncommon to find hyperthymesia coupled with obsessive personality traits, making the person systematically remember things even when it's not required. In the words of Jill Price, it is both a burden and a gift.

Every brain has the ability to remember such details, but we only utilise this ability when the day or event is particularly memorable, such as a wedding day or traumatic experience, when we are more aware of this sensory information.

This is due to how the brain prefers to store memories, because incredibly vivid details that are not experienced on a typical day are more easily remembered. Our memory can be trained to a limitless level, but it takes a strong imagination and a lot of repetition.

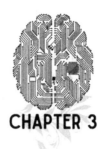

CHAPTER 3

The Future of Neuroscience

We can only see a short distance ahead, but we can see plenty there that needs to be done.

Alan Turing

This quote from Alan Turing, the famous World War II cryptanalyst and mathematician, summarises this chapter perfectly. We face so many challenges to achieve the future that we want and deserve, and it is perhaps our greatest strength that we can work together to solve each problem in order to get there. When we reflect on the past century and consider the progress we have made in health and medicine, technology and scientific experimentation, it is exciting to imagine what new frontiers may be open to us 100 years from now. This chapter will explore what that future could look like. Divided into three parts – science mixes with technology, health and disease, and enhancement – each one focuses on an element of our lives where progress in neuroscience is expected to have a big impact. It will serve as a guide through the most groundbreaking research today, and what exactly would be required for us to advance to a future where neuroscience could cure brain diseases or preserve our mind to live forever. It will talk about how we can unlock our brain's potential, one day communicating not with words, but with the power of our minds, and the research teams that are out there today trying to turn this into a reality.

It is a little over 50 years since we first landed astronauts on the Moon, and technology has developed at a radical rate in the years since. The computing power required for a three-man round trip to the Moon in 1969 could easily fit inside your smartphone today. In the coming century, technological advances may drive scientific discovery by helping us to look even closer at the brain, gaining unprecedented access to the body's most mysterious organ and driving us to a future that is less science fiction, and more science.

If you thought the brain was strange and mysterious before, just wait!

WE KNOW SO MUCH YET SO LITTLE

There are exciting times ahead of us in neuroscience, but it is essential to look at where we are today. There remains so much that we are yet to truly comprehend about the brain. It feels as though each time we learn something new many more questions arise to challenge our way of thinking about how the brain really works. For scientists to even comprehend what a human brain looks like, with its interconnecting neurons, axons, glial cells, blood vessels and neurotransmitters, we first need to construct a precise map, a *connectome*. Brain scans able to map a human brain in three dimensions, where we could trace each neuron to visualise the connections, would bring a revolutionary leap forwards that would rival mapping the human genome or landing on the Moon.

The human brain consists of billions of neurons, and thousands of synapses on each one. The first attempt to accurately map a small region of a fruit fly brain managed to capture around 600 neurons. At this rate, we need to combine that fly with another 146 million to even come close to the human brain. For this to happen, science would need to take an interdisciplinary approach where research is shared freely amongst other scientists, engineers, doctors and academics. This occurs much less than you might think, but some research institutions are beginning to change things. The Allen Institute in Seattle, USA, for example, does precisely that. They freely share their brain maps to help other researchers understand the workings of the brain and accelerate neuroscience as a whole. However, there remains an overwhelming demon that exists in the world of scientific publishing: the journals publishing the research charge an extortionate price to accept the research findings in the first place (thousands of dollars per research article) and then charge shameful subscription fees to grant access to them. This was famously highlighted when a Harvard University memo was released explaining how its $3.5 million yearly subscription bill was harming its scientific contribution.[1] It mentioned Elsevier, a Dutch publishing giant, which has a revenue of $2.6 billion, but the truth is they are only the tip of an increasingly large iceberg.

The response to the Covid-19 pandemic by some publishers is perhaps most concerning, which has resulted in price-gouging. The cost of some electronic books (digital copies with relatively small costs for publishing) has increased by up to 500% for students.[2] These books are often a course requirement. One example by McGraw Hill publishing showed a print edition for £65.99, but £528 for a downloadable version.

What all of this really means is that only the wealthiest establishments have access to all scientific research, but there is light at the end of the tunnel. The Indian government is considering a 'one nation one subscription' policy, through which it would buy the science articles and share them with scientists all over the country; an amazing idea that hopefully catches on. But globally, sadly, greed has crept its way into science, and if this greed goes unchallenged, greater connectivity between scientists will never be realised.

Let us assume that evil publishers do not exist for a moment, and let's get back to the fruit fly. Visual processing within its brain recruits around 60,000 neurons (the entire brain contains around 100,000). Let's say the fly sees a juicy apple in front of it – neurons from the visual cortex relay signals communicating with other brain regions, interpreting those signals to form a picture and determining that it is an apple. It turns out that only 10% of those neurons responded how we thought they should.[3] That leaves 90% of brain activation that we do not yet fully comprehend. Even that number is overly ambitious. We still do not understand how our brain uses different types of neurons to solve a problem. We have an idea, and can prove concepts, but not the entire story. Imagine reading a book missing some pages. If we read Goldilocks and the Three Bears, to see the heroine eating ice-cold porridge before falling asleep, missing the parts where she eats the warmer stuff, we would just think she was a strange porridge eater, used to Arctic conditions. We would lack the context we need.

There are many questions that will need answering if we want to advance into the future we envision. Despite the obstacles of scientific collaboration and publishing, ambitious biotechnology companies competing to be the first to establish themselves as leaders are partnering with academic researchers to bring the future closer than previously imaginable. Below I outline some of the most highly anticipated research in today's laboratories and how these projects are preparing to shape the future of neuroscience.

Part 1: Science mixes with technology

Imaging our brain

I must admit, when I first had the idea to write this chapter, my mind immediately went to 'Can my brain be transferred into a robot so I can live longer?' When I put out the call for people to submit neuroscience questions, I was reassured to see that other people were asking this question too. 'At least I won't be the only robot in the future,' I thought to myself. With that in mind, will it ever be possible to upload our memories, thoughts and personalities, into a computerised, synthetic brain, so that when our bodies die, we still have a version of ourselves that continues 'living'? If so, what would that look like, and how do we even start to create the technology? In the future, will we really have the skill to accomplish this?

Let's start with the idea of building a synthetic brain that would store all of our life experiences and personality. A computerised duplicate would need to be made where all of this information could be stored. One of the big milestones to making this future a reality is precisely scanning and mapping our brain. The human brain has 88–100 billion neurons, each with thousands, or tens of thousands, of synapses, meaning 1,000,000,000,000,000 connections to map (1 quadrillion). If we include brain cells that are not neurons, such as glial cells – for which we have up to five times as many as we do of neurons – it gets even more complicated, and don't even get me started on interneurons, a sort of go-between for two neurons. All of this will need to be mapped and visualised to understand and replicate a human brain. So, we just need a giant map then, right? Well... yes and no.

SEEING IS BELIEVING

One vital area that will see improvement within the next century is the technology that allows scientists to visualise what happens inside a neuron. Our most powerful microscopes, such as electron microscopes and two-photon microscopes (the latter is the gold-standard microscope, which involves firing a laser to light up or fluoresce neurons), require that the cells remain perfectly still, and therefore they cannot be alive. Living tissue can be imaged, but it generally results in slow pictures with less than ideal resolution.[a] However, imaging techniques that could visualise living brain cells in real time, such as observing how receptors and other proteins interact with medicines, would be a breakthrough that could allow us to see exactly how a drug works.

Newer and more specific imaging techniques that allow us to label or tag specific parts of brain cells would also enable researchers to track changes over time in multiple brain regions. We could essentially reverse engineer this information to understand what happens in the brain to start a disease process in the first place – processes that are difficult to study and still not fully explored. Today's microscopes have a trade-off between higher image quality with a slow processing time and frame rate, or a faster and deeper image with a lower resolution. Future imaging would need to blend both of these benefits while limiting the trade-offs. Alipasha Vaziri's New York-based research laboratory is currently attempting just that by developing a three-photon microscopy

---

[a] Improved two-photon microscopy by a US team working with live animals showed[4] impressive improvements using FACED (free space angular-chirp-enhanced delay), which records neurons with such a high frame rate as to be able to see the electrical signals. However, it only penetrates 1mm of brain tissue, and thus can't reach deeper areas.

technique that can take images much deeper than the standard 1mm.[b,5] They are able to record from 12,000 neurons simultaneously, all while the animal moves around and interacts with its environment, allowing researchers to study how the brain changes with its behaviour. This is truly an amazing accomplishment.

These big images would create so much data it could be difficult for standard computers to manage. Further improvements in these areas would therefore rely on joint innovation in technology, microscopy, computer software and artificial intelligence (AI) to process the information gathered from such images. It may be that advances in neuroscience will be coupled with these technological innovations.

In 2019, a research team at the Massachusetts Institute of Technology (MIT) paired up with Nobel-prize winning scientist Eric Betzig and his laboratory for a breathtaking look at neurons, where they decided to revisit the brain of – you guessed it – our favourite fruit fly.[6] They invented a technique called *expansion microscopy*, which basically means the neurons of the brain swell up in size to be able to create three-dimensional images. The images produced were revolutionary and allowed the researchers to zoom in on specific neurons and synapses, where they were able to count all 40 million synapses. That is incredible. It is like taking a picture of a needle in a haystack. Well, 40 million needles in a whole lot of haystacks. If those haystacks happened to fit on your fingertip.

Moving forward, this advanced microscopy could be coupled with virtual reality headsets to enable scientists to

[b] The research team is pioneering HyMS microscopy (hybrid multiplexed sculptured light microscopy) in live animal brains to see how they change as animals interact with their environment.

visualise all the brain connections (with use of a headset you could literally walk around the brain). Currently though, this technique has drawbacks, such as the specific parts of brain cells that do not fluoresce or don't like the swelling process. These issues will be addressed in further studies as we advance our understanding of these techniques.

CAN WE UPLOAD OUR MEMORIES?

So, back to building a computerised brain. The major issue with looking at human brain cells is that it tends to kill them in the process. The cells need to be stable and unable to move so we can get clear pictures in the laboratory (this is different to brain scans in a hospital that look at the entire brain, rather than just a few tiny neurons). One way around this problem, at least in today's laboratories, is to use the brains of the recently deceased. Another, more graphic way, is to wait until the moment a person is about to pass away, before preserving the brain. This will eventually be fatal, but the information will be gathered from a living brain, nonetheless. There is a company called Nectome doing just that. Terminally ill volunteers are choosing to have their brains preserved with the intention of storing their brain cells, and therefore their memories, in near perfect condition, essentially freezing their brain in time. Nectome is at the forefront of a brand new field of experimental neuroscience called memory preservation. In 2018, and just hours after death, a human brain was removed and preserved using Nectome's new technique. This proved the method worked.[7] The brain itself will be used for further studies into perfecting the storage process for others.

To do this new type of preservation, Nectome has developed a chemical solution based on glutaraldehyde to fix the brain and all of its microscopic structures in place for future generations to decode. This is no easy task when considering there are at least 300,000 molecules in each synapse, and we have no real idea as to which ones are functionally relevant in memories or how the cell uses them for long-term memory storage. Neuroscientists can already preserve brain tissue, but the process causes a lot of damage and would be nowhere near the level needed for a human brain to be of any use in the future. This is why Nectome's novel approach is so exciting.

The company's ambitious aim is to preserve brains ready for a time when they can be brought back to life in some form or another. However, many scientists believe that reanimating a human brain, even a century from now, is unrealistic. We still have little sense of how the brain is connected. Even if we have this connectome, this brain map will not necessarily be enough to teach us how to extract and decipher the brain's information. Nectome stress, however, that they are merely focusing on long-term preservation of brain tissue. They are dedicated to preserving the connections, synapses and axons that are the basis (at least as far as we know) for memory storage, and at this stage, they are not attempting to reanimate the brain.

Many questions around the specifics of memory formation remain unresolved and so it is unlikely that personality and behaviour could be identified and uploaded into a future avatar any time soon. Important questions remain frustratingly unanswered. If we think back to Chapter 1, where we explored the process of memory formation, one of the challenges of decoding memories is how small details about each memory are stored all over the brain. Connections to our emotional areas, visual areas, logical areas and so many more can make up a single memory. For example, would a single receptor or ion channel be responsible for remembering an instance when you once laughed at a joke, or for feelings of empathy you once had for a loved one, or cherishing a painting you once saw? Even more intriguing – if we understand these changes could we delete memories that we *don't* want? You may want to remember a happy experience at a theme park, for example, but not the part where you throw up after a ride.

What is more plausible is that we will learn to 'read' some of the brain's data at a basic level, such as what decade the memories are from, what language a person spoke or a vague description of a location previously visited. This is more challenging than it sounds because a single memory is not stored as a movie reel or a picture: instead, it consists of a collection of details from neuronal interactions, each with their own subtle changes. Decoding this connectome would require powerful AI to learn not only *how* the brain cells are connected, but *why* they are connected. To solve this problem, a wireless headset worn by the person, coupled to advanced AI, could be used for months before the brain undergoes the preservation process. This would be crucial when decoding the connectome to reanimate the brain pathways in a synthetic brain or to 'restart' the original organic brain.

Suppose it is possible to retrieve memories from a deceased brain. Depending on how long the brain has been dead, it may be possible to upload our memories post mortem, potentially to solve crimes using the last memories before a murder. Or perhaps we may one day download memories from living people, using a wireless device to see the truth in a criminal trial. Eventually, the consumer market will utilise this technology, and with it, create a future in which we could recall our own memories at will, using a wireless device to identify a happy memory, directions to a location once visited or a simple shopping list.

Future neuroscience investigations and products would almost certainly move in the direction of non-invasive recording. Today, our most reliable data come from electrodes surgically implanted into the brain. Often, studies will recruit people who have electrode implants to treat epileptic seizures to minimise invasive procedures on people who do not need them. Still, we are slowly moving to a future that could detect brain changes wirelessly, as we will see below.

SAME HEAD, NEW BODY

If we want to preserve our brain, can't we just cut out the middle-man, quite literally? Why bother going through all the effort of uploading and decoding our brain when we die, when we could just transplant our head onto another, healthy body.

Pause for the reader to throw up.

In 1908, a scientist named Charles Guthrie attempted to put the head of one dog onto the neck of another. It didn't live more than a few hours. Fast forward to 1971, however, and a team of surgeons carried out a gruesome transplantation of a monkey's head onto another monkey's body. The monkey survived for 8 days and the surgeons actually managed to restore some basic sensations such as smell, taste and hearing.[8] Of course, this is the stuff of nightmares and a reminder of the sacrifices that are, sadly, made in the name of science. Then, in 2019, a 33-year-old Russian man named Valery Spiridonov, suffering from a muscle-wasting disease, was set to become the first human to undergo a full head transplant onto another's body. In the years leading up to the potential surgery, he had joined up with Italian neurosurgeon Sergio Canavero to perform the world's first human head transplant. Spiridonov recently removed himself as a volunteer for the surgery, however, after marrying his partner and deciding against the risky procedure. Science is clearly determined to prove the feasibility of this type of surgery, as Canavero is committed to finding another volunteer in the future.

Aside from the ethical considerations of this kind of operation (Canavero has difficulties in performing his research in many countries for this reason), the technical capabilities needed to achieve it are far beyond our reach today. Understanding how to reattach a spinal cord and its neurons, or preserve blood flow to the body and brain, or how to combine many surgical skills for the neck, blood vessels, nerves and everything else, are all challenges that most do not believe we are capable of solving any time soon.

BRAIN-COMPUTER INTERFACES

One of the most thrilling ideas to come from blending neuroscience and engineering together is one that will have the greatest influence on how we live our lives in the future. Called brain–computer interfaces, or BCIs, they create a direct communication between the human brain and a computer. Simply by using the power of our thoughts, we can interact with the world around us in a completely new way. In fact, research of this type has been continually improving since the 1970s, and now we are finally starting to see the benefit from this technology and where its potential may be. This area is growing at such a rapid rate that the BCI consumer market is expected to be worth $4 billion by 2027.

Virtual reality is already with us, and anyone who owns a games console has likely seen the equipment advertised somewhere. They range from a small headset with a smartphone inserted, to a fully immersive racing car game where every angle you view provides you with a realistic feeling of driving outside. Now, Neurable, a company in Boston, USA, has moved us one step closer to the ultimate experience by showcasing its virtual reality game, called Awakening. What is different about this game is that the movement through this virtual reality is controlled with your mind. Other companies such as Nextmind also want to pair cutting-edge neuroscience with new technology to create products like this for the public. It has developed a headset that analyses a person's eye movement and translates it into a command. For instance, if the headset is worn while watching TV it can change the channel, increase the volume and open up menu screens. It is available for public purchase today, but this is only the first step in BCI development.

Several companies, such as Brainco, Neurosity, Paradromics and Neurable, are figuring out ways to better record and monitor electrodes in the brain. Currently, the most precise measurements from our brain come from surgically implanted electrodes that burrow into the brain itself. Of course, this will not be great for use in the general public, and today this method is reserved only for people with severe brain disorders that cannot be treated in other ways. Electrodes can be as small as a human hair in an attempt to minimise damage to the brain itself. Wireless EEG devices are in development and will be the direction this technology follows in the future, eventually miniaturising to a size unnoticeable by those around you. Several BCIs that utilise standard EEG measurements are currently on the market, advertised as helping with meditation, attention levels, sleep and emotional states. For recording brain signals, the middle ground between high-sensitivity recording with electrodes or non-invasive techniques with low sensitivity is being studied by a company called Synchron. In 2020 it successfully inserted electrodes through the jugular vein in the neck, enabling two patients with motor neuron disease, who were incapable of moving, to communicate via text message.[9] It involved AI software spending weeks learning their brain signals before picking out selected words only by the person thinking them. This is important because it suggests that greater detection of brain signals can be accomplished without having to insert electrodes into the brain, and although this may only find potential in medical circumstances, rather than consumer products, future studies are already looking to improve electrode recording devices. Any electrode will always cause brain cell damage, and although the initial surgery for implantation is relatively safe, we do not understand the long-term damage caused by implanted electrodes. Newer recording devices that can measure brain signals perfectly without causing cell damage would overcome that.

WRITE LIKE A COMPUTER

In 2017 Facebook boldly claimed that it would create a wearable device that could transform your thoughts into words at an impressive speed, attempting to type 100 words per minute (the average is 40). Facebook's Reality Labs are partnering with several research teams across universities to develop an AI system that can translate a person's thoughts into text by analysing their brain activity. So far, one team has created AI to recognise 250 words, although presently they are selected from pre-chosen sentences – a far stretch from real conversation. A decade after speech was first decoded from brain activity, this technology is still in its infancy, but Facebook predicts that within the next 10 years, we will start to see more impressive developments from this research. Reality Labs say that this is likely to come in the form of augmented reality glasses. They want to use light to measure oxygen levels in the brain, instead of invasive brain electrodes. This works because the more activity there is in the brain, the more oxygen it uses, which can be observed. It uses a similar method to MRI scans, which measure increased blood flow to parts of the brain. Although there is a lot of development required, it is reassuring to see how neuroscience is linked with cutting-edge technology. This drive for consumer products is also helping to advance our understanding of how the brain works and how it turns an electrical signal into an action.

The potential for this technology will surely see it integrated into our homes the same way that Amazon's Alexa is used at the moment. We could be ordering our local takeout food just by using a headset to convert our thoughts into choices from the menu. Consumer BCIs would see products similar to today's fitness trackers, worn by millions, eventually becoming integrated into everyday life. The future of BCIs for the public will see them used in augmented reality devices for everything from social media, shopping or interacting with ordinary objects in the street. Although the devices may be seen as commonplace in the future, the neuroscience principles they are based on have been a subject of study for over a century.

Those principles have been taken to a new level by a team in Helsinki, Finland. Artificial intelligence, hooked up to EEG devices from 31 people, was able to learn what the people were seeing.[10] This AI learning is what scientists call *neuroadaptive generative modelling* (scientists seem to enjoy making up these impressively long names). The volunteers looked at certain faces or people smiling, old or young, male or female, and over time the AI learned to interpret those signals. That isn't all though. It didn't just learn to read those signals, it started to interpret them and form its own image of what the people were seeing. It created brand new pictures of what it thought the volunteers might be looking at. This is impressive, because if we want to create a future where we learn to decode the brain's information, AI machine learning will have to play a crucial part. This experiment demonstrates to some extent just how close we are to achieving that, even if only at a basic level for now.

COMMUNICATION

We have seen the first signs that neuroscience will benefit communication. In practical terms, neuroscience offers a unique chance to help people communicate who may not have the ability to do so independently. We have the science today for people who cannot talk or move any part of their body to communicate by slowly picking letters, or pre-chosen words, using eye movements. As great as that is, we can do better. Looking ahead, there is a great deal of potential for improvement.

If converting your thoughts into a computerised voice is slow, why not just skip the voice, and go straight into the other person's brain? In 2019, brain-to-brain communication was realised by Andrea Stocco at the University of Washington in Seattle, who had two volunteers watch light at either 15Hz or 17Hz.[11] Previously, it has been shown that if we hook up the brain to an EEG, we can observe differences in how the brain responds to the different frequencies of light. In the experiment, when the two people looked at the 15Hz light, it was detected by the EEG placed onto the head and converted into a signal through a local computer connection. This message was then sent to another room, where a third person had that electrical signal sent directly to their brain. If the signal was 15Hz, then the third person would see a flash of light (their brain activity makes this happen). If it was 17Hz, there would be no light. This technique is still very new but what it shows is that your brainwaves can be transmitted to another area and decoded into a message. Currently, this message will be the equivalent of a binary code (1s and 0s), which is not particularly exciting, but it means that silent communication between people in different locations is possible. In this experiment, seeing a flash of light would be a 1 and seeing no light would be a 0. All with only the mind. Theoretically, there wouldn't be a limit to the distance that this signal could be sent over, meaning that global communication could happen. You could be sitting through a boring meeting but silently messaging your friend about dinner plans with your boss none the wiser, provided your friend understands binary code. If neuroscientists can categorise the meaning behind different brainwaves then eventually this could feed into virtual reality headsets, where the internet, for example, could be explored with only our thoughts. You could walk around the internet while sitting on your couch. Of course, this is a distant future, but the science tells us that it will be possible some day.

This experiment demonstrated that it is possible to send a basic signal to one person, but in the future, communication between hundreds of people, simultaneously, could be achieved. Teaching, business meetings and social events could all be established through these experimental concepts, although for a full consumer product it would likely take much longer to produce than laboratory studies. People will have to learn to accept this new technology, and high-resolution, non-invasive (i.e. not using electrodes, but headsets instead) products would need to be shown to be safe, reliable, and affordable for this to become a reality. I really hope it does.

LANGUAGE

If speaking with your mind to another person isn't enough, Microsoft has developed the technology to translate 70 languages in real time for face-to-face conversations. The Microsoft Translator app is the first stage in developing a universal translator, but already it can allow 100 people to join a conversation (limited to one person speaking at a time). Considering the translator learns more than one million words for each language (keep in mind that one person's vocabulary is only around 20,000 words), it is a strong starting point for future universal communicators. Progress within this area would see the translations happen within our own brains, without the need for an external device to translate what was spoken. If brain-to-brain communication continues to advance along the same trajectory as it is predicted, then this translation could occur imperceptibly fast within our own thoughts. You could actually hear someone else talking inside your head (although that sounds quite horrifying at first). If you are not quite ready for having different voices in your brain, then don't worry. Next generations of translators will probably be integrated into some sort of wearable device, like glasses or an earpiece, but the prospect of BCIs pairing with language translators is fascinating.

On a side note, as great as it is talking with other people, it has long been a dream of humans to communicate with animals. A company called Zoolingua currently believes that its invention to communicate with dogs is less than 10 years away. Observing the dogs through video footage, it believes that it can decipher each bark and sound into a meaningful translation. Considering that 70% of pet owners say that they can clearly understand their own pet's forms of communication, we may see pet translation devices reasonably soon. That said, there is currently much that we do not know about communication between animals, particularly about their language centres in the brain. Speech and language centres in human brains are highly developed, and translating our knowledge of the human brain into those of other animals has generally proven to be unreliable.

As dogs primarily communicate through body language and use a more basic form of communication than humans, a North Carolina State University group has created a harness-mounted computer with sensors that monitor and decode the dog's emotional state. Although this may not be of much use for regular pet owners, there is a push for this technology to help train search and rescue, bomb-sniffing and service dogs. If technology and science continue to develop, wearable devices would be a strong basis to connect human and animal minds. This may not involve communicating directly, but rather sharing some basic emotional responses.

PART II: HEALTH AND DISEASE

ORGANOIDS

Historically, for neuroscientists to learn how different brain regions worked and why they were important, they relied upon observing the outcome of brain injuries. These injuries would result in some form of limited brain function, with scientists often damaging specific areas in animals to observe the effect (the 20th century saw some very questionable ethics). Other experimental techniques relied on changing how brain cells work by adding drugs to increase or decrease brain function. Future research will depend on scientific investment into better models of disease. Models are, essentially, experiments set up in a laboratory to test treatments before they ever get near a patient.

Of course, scientists rely on models in research today, but what we really need are experiments showing the start of the disease. This is extremely difficult to study in people. By the time neurological symptoms appear, the disease has already advanced, so scientists are looking at new ways to model the disease's early phases. By understanding the *pathogenesis* of a disease (how it develops), future medical care can focus on markers of the start of a disease. The markers could be specific proteins that are released in the body which signal that the disease is developing. It is these *biomarkers* that could change the shape of how we screen and detect neurological disorders early. Although scientists can find lots of changes in a patient's blood (typically where we would look for biomarkers) they often don't correlate very well with the early stages of disease. This is why we need a better look at what happens, so we can find new ones.

With advancements in models like organoids, which we are about to explore, we will enter a new age of discovery of disease-specific biomarkers, helping diagnose and treat diseases more accurately than ever before.

Brain organoids will bring a new way of understanding more about diseases, and neuroscientists are already using them to learn more about the brain and the pathogenesis of disease. Brain organoids are groups of stem cells grown in a laboratory that change into different types of cells, forming a three-dimensional kind of mini-brain. In today's laboratories, they are too simplistic to resemble a human brain, as they lack blood vessels and an immune system, but organoids do have some of the critical features needed to study the brain. For example, scientists can look at how individual cell types interact with one another to give unprecedented insights into cell systems.[12] By observing organoid cells' life cycle researchers can gain a deeper understanding of how diseases develop.

For example, a team of researchers at Harvard Medical School has created an organoid that mimics Alzheimer's disease and looks at how the Aβ peptide (amyloid beta), a key part of the disease, is produced and accumulates inside cells.[a] The team believes that this type of organoid could lead to the discovery of future biomarkers and novel tests for other genetic diseases.

Organoids may be especially important in psychiatric disorders like schizophrenia, where results from experiments using animal models are difficult to apply to humans. As of yet, experimental models are not equipped to give us the detail we

---

[a] Mutations in the *APP* (amyloid precursor protein) and *PSEN1* (presenilin 1) genes were looked at specifically because they are known to be risk factors for developing Alzheimer's disease.[13]

need to translate that to human brains, but we are getting closer to a human brain model. Organoids are a relatively new aspect of neuroscience research, but future organoids that combine techniques such as tissue engineering with synthetic biology, where nanotechnology could be introduced into living cells, would be a powerful future direction for this technique.

Scientists could use this combination of technologies to observe and record cell processes, such as how transport mechanisms along the brain cell develop and malfunction, or what cellular changes result in long-term memory. If, say, human-made scaffolds or programmed viruses could be used to help neurons find others to form new connections, an improved organoid system could be used to study what that looks like. For example, a study from 2020 showed how the herpes virus can directly produce a new organoid system for Alzheimer's disease, which has many of the features of the real disease in humans.[14] Maybe next time, you'll feel a bit more admiration for that cold sore on your mouth.

These studies will undoubtedly lead to major improvements in protecting against neuronal loss in stroke, dementia and cancer. Actually, this technology is already filtering in, as nanomedicine can now use 3D arrangements of cells to customise their configuration to how scientists want them, using a technique called DPAC (DNA-programmed assembly of cells). Basically, it is a long way of explaining how scientists can control the shape of 3D cellular structures. It has the potential to create thousands of tiny organoids at one time, which have the ability to stick to each other like Velcro and create more extensive 'brain-like' cultures.[15] Think of DPAC organoids as being like Lego bricks that are assembled to create a bigger Lego brain. This will help scientists to get even closer to creating an entire brain region in the laboratory, which could be used for drug screening, teaching and learning, and partial transplants in the coming century.

Nanomedicine is going even further and beginning to utilise scaffolds made of graphene, a carbon material with the thickness of just one single atom that can be shaped in a way to allow laboratory-grown cells to develop in a more precise way, like an even smaller and more specialised Lego block. Cells grown three-dimensionally (rather than two-dimensionally on a flat dish) will better mimic the real human body. Graphene scaffolds are particularly interesting because they can be placed back into the body, with the cells attached, to promote normal cell growth. Scientists hope that they can help repair spinal cord and brain cells, which today is an incredibly complex challenge. This would dramatically change the outcome for patients who have lost sensation to parts of their body through spinal cord trauma and can't walk, or those who have experienced trauma to the brain, resulting in cell death and impacting their speech, movement or memories. It could have a significant influence on the lives of many people medicine is still struggling to treat.

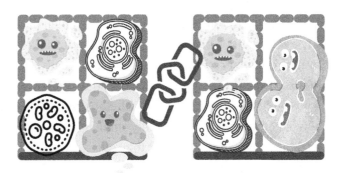

By linking cells together just the way scientists want, it opens up a whole new level of experimental design. One which gets scientists closer to creating the real thing, a real brain to learn from.

CRISPR

One of the purest motivations for medicine would be to improve our standards of health and allow us to live longer and happier lives – a simple idea, but one with complicated challenges. Our brain can do extraordinary things, but with this ability comes a greater risk of errors. Diseases affecting the brain during our lifetime eventually will be preventable or reversible to the extent that we may live with an improved quality of life almost indistinguishable from that of someone with a healthy brain.

Neurodegeneration[b] of our brain cells, as seen in Alzheimer's, Parkinson's and Huntington's diseases, is an area desperately in need of new and innovative treatments.

There are hundreds of clinical trials underway for neurodegeneration, but because so many trials fail in humans, we rarely see a patient benefit from them. Typically, clinical trials for neurodegeneration can take up to two years to prove any benefit. Although we like to imagine that a patient will recover immediately with clear and obvious improvements, the trial will commonly establish only small improvements in cognitive ability, which take longer to prove.

However, the future of medical treatments does look promising. Although it has been more than 18 years since the USA last approved a new drug for Alzheimer's disease, we are now closer than ever to a new generation of treatments. Biogen's monoclonal antibody aducanumab has been shown to slow the progression of the disease[16] and although its effects are very limited, it represents a big step forward in our approach to slowing down disease progression – an encouraging sign for the near future. With this in mind, therapies that slow the progression of the disease will soon start to surface, aiming to give people extra precious years of relatively normal life.[c] Subtle differences in the genetics of neurological disorders mean that it may be more challenging

---

[b] Neurodegeneration is the term for when cells of the central nervous system (brain and spinal cord) lose their function and structure and fail to work as they should.

[c] BIIB092 (gosuranemab) and RO7105705 (semorinemab) are IgG4 anti-tau antibodies currently the subjects of some of the most promising clinical trials, with evidence of up to a 96% reduction in tau within the cerebrospinal fluid. Tau is a protein found in neurons and helps with cell signalling, plasticity and regulating genes. However, once it is created, it can change its shape and cause harm inside the neuron. When tau molecules clump together they can eventually lead to neuronal death.

to produce similar responses in every patient; new-generation treatments are more likely to focus on subsets of patients with specific genetic components to the disease that can be targeted more precisely, and with better results (a tactic known as personalised medicine).

The idea of taking a few pills and waiting for the benefits to roll through is probably coming to the end of its lifespan, and the development of future treatments will undoubtedly utilise new technologies that are showing promising results even today. So, what would that look like?

In 2012, Emmanuelle Charpentier and her research team demonstrated that a small piece of RNA (the genetic blueprint for building proteins) could be constructed in a way as to guide a specific protein[d] to a particular DNA sequence.[17] This is important because this isn't just any old protein. It is one that cuts the DNA strand in our cells, so that it no longer looks like the familiar double helix – instead, some parts are now floating freely. When the body notices that DNA is not in its usual double helix, repair mechanisms are triggered. Normally, this keeps our DNA in good working order. This process of repair actually happens every day of our lives. We don't even have to do anything, we can just kick back and relax and let our body do the rest.

A technique called CRISPR, short for Clustered Regularly Interspaced Short Palindromic Repeats, takes advantage of the fact that this repair mechanism is far from perfect, and is prone to introducing errors. Sometimes, this causes the body to produce a faulty DNA sequence that stops that section, or gene, from working. CRISPR is a powerful tool if you want to

---

[d] The most widely used protein, Cas9, was adapted from bacterial defences against viruses and other pathogens, whereby they would cut foreign DNA apart to halt the attack.

stop an already 'faulty' gene or prevent a gene from working, allowing scientists to observe the effects. CRISPR can even introduce new genes. For example, it could be used in plants and animals to increase resistance to environmental factors such as drought or potentially remove malaria-carrying mosquitoes' capacity to reproduce.

The most exciting use of CRISPR could be to expand our range of experimental tools to understand the impact of genes on neurological diseases and why those diseases first appear. This exciting prospect of a future with CRISPR has scientists gleefully rubbing their hands together in anticipation. If you ever notice a scientist doing this, now you know what they are thinking about. By learning more about how genetic mutations lead to diseases like Parkinson's and Alzheimer's, we could see advancements in treatments sooner than previously thought. Future therapies may focus on reversing an already present illness or preventing it from ever occurring by repairing the genes that lead to the disease.[e,18] To show this, Birgitt Schüle's research team in the USA grew some stem cells and corrected the DNA damage typically seen in Parkinson's disease.[19] The idea is that the stem cells would be infused back into the patient as a sort of stem cell replacement therapy.

[e] Several genetic defects are being targeted by CRISPR methods, such as cystic fibrosis, cataracts and Fanconi anaemia, but this is only at the experimental stage as of yet. Research teams are also attempting to use CRISPR to target bacterial and viral infections with the hope of finding a common RNA sequence on which to base a universal therapy.

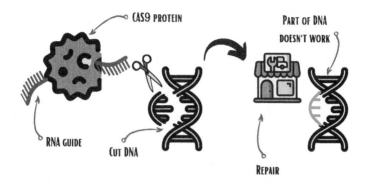

CRISPR is a gene-editing tool. By introducing cuts at precise locations in the DNA, the repair mechanisms can result in stopping a gene from working.

A similar method has also received optimism for Alzheimer's disease after stem cells were reprogrammed to make them resistant to the disease and age-related cognitive decline.[20] This new style of gene therapy is also applicable to other conditions. A research team in the USA has edited stem cells to correct for a gene mutation involved in cystic fibrosis,[21] and genes for a specific type of anaemia were altered by scientists as part of an international research effort between two groups in the USA and Germany.[22]

Within the turn of the century, this technique will routinely be used to alter genetic codes for those who are most at risk of developing neurodegenerative diseases.[23] Of course, the ethical implications are enormous and should be carefully considered, but the scientific capabilities are still amazing.

The prospects for CRISPR's future are thrilling, and in fact, clinical trials are already underway to alter immune cells outside of the patient's body, programming them to fight cancer.[f,24] One reason we will use it in the future is the low cost and relative simplicity, which will ensure that more research groups, particularly in less well-funded laboratories, can develop the technique for treating other diseases. A greater variety of research groups that replicate existing data will improve the speed at which we see CRISPR utilised for future treatments. Given that only five years after the introduction of CRISPR scientists claimed to have already used it to remove heart defects in an embryo,[g,25] the future of treating neurological diseases may rest in genetic manipulation.

Using CRISPR is undoubtedly going to be important in the future of neuroscience, but there are unresolved issues that limit its potential use, which research in today's laboratories is trying to address. A novel technology comes with novel challenges, and the precision of the repair mechanisms is not as good as scientists would like. Initially, the best results only offered around 80% efficiency, meaning that it doesn't work as intended 20% of the time. This would rule out most uses for human diseases, but as the technology develops, so will the specificity and efficiency. This was already shown by a group of scientists in 2018, when CRISPR reached a new level. By analysing thousands of pieces of DNA, and billions of potential combinations, scientists were able to develop a method of

---

[f] CRISPR is being used to engineer patient T cells (crucial immune cells that kill infected cells, and stimulate B cells to make antibodies) to express a new receptor recognising cancer cells. The engineered immune cells are then replaced in patients' blood, and we are seeing high success rates. Further to this, rodent studies in which scientists remove the gene responsible for suppressing T cells have resulted in increased T cell counts and decreased tumour size. The research team aims to use this intervention early in cancer to maintain high T cell levels in patients.

[g] An international effort produced this data although some scientists doubt its credibility and say that the bad DNA was not corrected, but instead removed entirely.[26]

predicting precisely which sequences should be targeted for improving efficiency, meaning fewer errors and greater reliability.[27] Future, here we come!

Another challenge is that the protein itself, the one that cuts the DNA, is relatively large and thus finding its way into the nucleus of a cell (where the changes are made) is difficult. Commonly they are packed into a virus (perfectly safe to use at this point) because viruses are designed for one thing, which is to get to the nucleus of a cell. The problem is that the size limits the number of genes that can be edited at any time, and improving this delivery is what scientists have been trying to achieve. Thankfully, they didn't have to wait long to see an improvement. A research team recently showed how multiple genes could be edited at one time (editing up to 25).[28] Although more genes will need to be edited than just 25, potentially hundreds, it shows that scientists are heading in the right direction and are approaching the challenges with optimism and creativity. It strongly suggests that in the future, more genes will be targeted and with greater efficiency, and we will see a new generation of therapies benefiting from gene-editing techniques.

STAR TREK

So, if we can model diseases better within a laboratory, and use new imaging techniques, what would that actually look like? Could this technology be miniaturised and used by patients without the need for hospital visits? Will we ever see a future in which we use hand-held scanners similar to those used in the famous TV show *Star Trek*? Well, the short answer is yes.

In 2012 Qualcomm sponsored a multimillion-dollar 'XPrize' to bring the Star Trek tricorder to life. In the popular sci-fi TV show, this tricorder could be used to scan the DNA of alien life forms, diagnose a multitude of diseases and injuries, and even analyse elements in the atmosphere. Thanks to this prize fund, Basil Leaf Technologies has unveiled its DxtER AI-driven prototype.[29] Although much larger in size than that of the TV show, it can fit onto a tablet or smartphone and is equipped with a digital stethoscope, wrist and chest sensors, blood pressure and glucose monitors, amongst other features. It can even guide a user to provide a urine sample for laboratory testing if necessary. What is most impressive is that, just like the Star Trek scanner, all the tests are non-invasive.

Although the individual tests are readily available in any hospital, future medical care could see all-in-one scanners like this one as commonplace. Being able to have all of these tests available in one piece of equipment would help people to reach a diagnosis and treatment faster, especially in rural areas far away from hospitals. Within the next decades, the use of AI for automated responses and virtual reality hospital visits could see many laboratory tests replaced with home-kit style scanners. The results would be sent to the doctor, and if needed, further testing and observation in a hospital setting could be offered. Today's scanner has the potential to detect infections, diabetes, heart issues, breathing problems and high blood pressure, and it can even use a special non-invasive blood test (that's right, no blood draw needed). In the future, this could also be directed towards brain health by detecting novel biomarkers for neurological diseases.

The scanners wouldn't be intended to replace a qualified doctor in a hospital but could be useful in early detection of diseases and long-term clinical trials, whereby the patient can remain at home without the need for frequent trial centre visits. Coupled with other aspects of neuroscience advances, such as advanced imaging, they could drastically change how we think about health screenings in the future.

Part III: Enhancement

Into the Matrix

If neuroscience research is increasingly leading scientists to collaborate with pioneering technology companies, then why stop at virtual reality headsets and *Star Trek* scanners? Would it ever be possible to use our knowledge of the brain to enhance ourselves? We could not only make ourselves superhuman, but also help people who have suffered irreversible damage and are forced to live a more limited life.

Much of this chapter has focused on how neuroscience can improve our health, increase our life span or help people with life-altering issues. This section is all about how our understanding of the brain can enhance us and improve us beyond our natural capabilities. One thing that comes to mind when thinking about the enhancement of our brains is the movie *The Matrix*. For those of you who haven't seen it, the film revolves around a character called Neo who comes to realise that he is living in a digital world, the Matrix, and needs to be 'woken up' to go back to reality. At one point in the film, he goes into a sort of practice Matrix, where his mind can be uploaded with anything he wants, such as learning kung fu or how to use weapons. This happens within seconds, and his brain now has the 'muscle memory' for using these skills inside the Matrix. Is there a way to teach the brain to form memories on their own, without having to go through the long process of actually acquiring experience? Well sort of, yes.

In one of the most impressive studies so far in this book, and one that, at least in my mind, was carried out with lightning storms in a gothic castle somewhere, a rat was able to transfer its experience of going through a maze to another rat, saving him the effort of learning it for himself.[30] For anonymity, the names of the rats have been changed.

A rat (Pinky) had to perform a task that involved pulling levers, walking through a maze and interacting with things along the way. When he did this, the brain signals were transmitted into another rat (The Brain) who was relaxing elsewhere, unaware of Pinky's tasks. Scientists found that he learned everything much quicker, especially the maze. He still needed a few attempts, but not as many as Pinky did on his first run. It won't be long before they are working together to take over the world.

This suggests that information is encoded, at least partly, the same way in different brains and that the brain learns to respond to things even if we just 'pretend' to see it. This study also helped us to learn a lot about how much the brain relies on touch and sight to process information. Think about it as if you are about to take a test and your friend gives you the answer sheet before you take it. The answer sheet doesn't have everything written perfectly for you, but it does give you the first parts of what you need, and lots of hints. This gets you going and removes a lot of the lag time you need to create the answers for yourself. Precisely why the full amount of learning cannot be transmitted, or in this scenario, why the answer sheet isn't complete, we don't know. The potential for this is awesome. It may be possible in the future to choose something that we want to learn, and essentially, expose our brain to those same instructions. We could even do this while the brain is at rest, during a sleep state, where our brains are consolidating memories and new information that we were exposed to during the day. In theory, this is not a radical idea. Our brain can benefit from activities without ever doing them. Visualisation techniques, like positive thinking and rehearsing scenarios in your mind, have already been demonstrated to have a big impact on performance in sports.[31] One study was even able to show how visualisation could lead to an increase in brain signals to muscles, without actually moving them, leading to improved muscle strength in fingers and the elbow.[32] Advancing the research in this field would undoubtedly lead to some amazing changes in how we learn and improve.

Just imagine walking into the nearest Brainskills store, picking a USB stick from the shelf to help learn Mandarin or Spanish, and plugging it into your headset while relaxing on a beach somewhere. We may not learn the language entirely, but the next time we try to speak, it would seem more familiar to us, and with practice, those familiar memories would be formed into long-term memories of the language. It would give new meaning to a weekend of binging on Netflix or Brainskills TV.

PROSTHETICS

Scientists are now looking to build implantable components for our brain, to restore brain function after damage occurs. The Hippocampus Rebuild Project from two research teams in the US has made an exciting leap forward in this direction.[33] They were able to use a person's own memory patterns to reinforce natural memory encoding and recall, like having backup singers for the headline artist. They are singing the same song, but making it more powerful and, essentially, ensuring that the brain encodes the information into a sustainable and robust memory, easily remembered.

In the study, epilepsy patients had electrodes inserted into their hippocampus to study episodic memory, the type of memory used to remember useful information. The participants performed memory tasks, and the electrical firing patterns were recorded, analysed and 'started singing' back to the neurons when the task was repeated. There was an immediate improvement, with participants now able to remember 37% more. This is a fantastic achievement and a promising sign that we are successfully developing our understanding of how memories are created and how we can treat disorders in the future. Treatment for memory loss from dementia, stroke and brain injuries will benefit from studies like this.

However, there is a long way to go. Currently, this is only memory reinforcement and not the creation of new memories, which we are many years away from achieving. Even so, the potential implications are exciting. Eventually we could technically create new memories, either fictional or real, to bring stories and cinema to life, or to recover lost memories as a result of disease and cognitive decline.

Research is currently underway to build a prosthetic eye made from the same material that is used in solar cells. When light hits our eyes, it stimulates our retina at the back of our eye. This area is coated with millions of light-sensitive cells that convert the light into a signal that travels along the optic nerve into the brain. The idea behind this research is that by using perovskite, the conductive and light-sensitive material from solar cells, scientists can create tiny nanowires that mimic the cells along the retina. What is really fascinating, is because perovskite wires are so small, the density of the prosthetic retina cells is incredibly high – even higher than in the human eye. The artificial retina is still undergoing further development but it may not be long before enhancements such as these are available.

FINAL THOUGHT

Although it may seem strange or ridiculous today, the potential for neuroscience to change our future is real. Imagine synthetic material on the nanometer scale, able to stimulate the release of brain chemicals to promote our own brain neurogenesis (growth of new neurons). Material that will be programmed to work only on specific neurons (by injecting into the area of the brain we want) by identifying a particular part of the neuron. The growth of neurons could be targeted in the spinal cord or motor neurons, enabling people to move freely, or in the visual cortex to cure certain types of blindness.

The ethical considerations are huge for all of it. This future could launch humans into the next stage of our legacy, but just because we *can* change our DNA, improve our health or enhance our minds, it doesn't mean that we *should*. Consider the embryo, the little squidgy ball of cells just floating around minding its own business before becoming a person. We could improve any inevitable diseases before they develop, but we clearly don't have the consent of this future person. Early intervention will focus on preventing life-changing issues, but the relentless pursuit of better scientific understanding will bring with it the ability to alter many aspects of a person. Almost like a sort of menu, where you can pick and choose how you want your child to be, how they develop or what they will look like.

If science can alter genes to prevent diseases, could they also change genes to alter personality? If you had the choice would you decide to be born as a better athlete, or with a better memory, or be a more determined person?

If these choices do become available, at what point do we consider consent? It would never be possible to ask permission from an unborn baby. What if they would never have wanted to be changed, even if it is for an overall benefit?

With the advances in technology allowing people to gain a better insight into how the brain responds to different situations, in learning and memory for example, how would this change how we learn? Would schools and universities be different? Would you want your brain activity monitored to assess your attention levels to be compared with your fellow classmates? If this becomes a routine method of advanced teaching, how safe would your mind really be? Would your personal brain data be safe, or could someone intentionally alter your activity?

The future of neuroscience will bring with it a promise for a better life, improved health and a sense of control over our own mind. We should never fear the unknown but we should respect it, as it brings with it questions that will scratch at the deepest levels of our conscience.

You will have to answer some of those questions for yourself before we can step into this future.

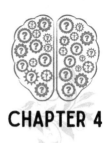

CHAPTER 4

DOWN THE SCIENCE RABBIT HOLE

INTRODUCTION

Now that you have all of this expert knowledge about the brain, what do you do with it? If you read about a particular idea that piqued your interest or encouraged your curiosity, then we are about to take a look at some ways in which you can develop that. This chapter will explore how science infiltrates all parts of our lives and just how easy it can be to get more involved. It will explain how you can turn your natural curiosity into something more real, regardless of how technical you want to get.

It will describe how having a scientific background can open up a bigger world for you, which may surprise even the most seasoned scientist. It could be that you have enjoyed this book and want to see what else is out there for you to explore. Or maybe you are currently on your path to becoming a scientist through advanced education. This chapter will have something for everyone as we discuss how your unique talents and skills can be poured into many different aspects of science. Whether this is the first science book you've read or it's number 257 currently sitting on a pile inside your book castle, I want to share with you some of the more hidden ways in which you can use and develop your nose for science in some creative and unusual ways.

It may be a little off topic from the core neuroscience I've focused on in the rest of the book, but now that you have a good understanding of what the brain does, and how scientists study it, I want to discuss what else scientists can do. There is a whole other side to the beast that is science. Sure, there are nerds in lab coats running experiments to create the next monster for a Frankenstein novel, but what happens when the monster is created? How does that monster then integrate itself into everyday life, or to put it another way, what scientific professions are there to help keep the cogs turning in society? From clinical trials to filing patents on new revolutionary products, to selling them to the people who need them, or perhaps even showing up on TV to talk about them. Sounds intriguing? Great! Because we are about to explore what all of that means, and how your knowledge of science can add an extra level of pizazz to your life.

I'M NOT A SCIENTIST BUT I WANT TO LEARN MORE

In this section, we will talk a little about how you can take your new knowledge of the brain and keep going. How you can expand on what you have learned to keep going down the rabbit hole of ever more exciting science stuff. You don't need a science background to keep learning more – there are a ton of ways in which you can do it. The trick is to find out what interests you the most. This won't be the same for everybody – it will be unique to you. Maybe it is rare brain diseases, or the history of neuroscience, or perhaps the future? Even if you have only 10 minutes on a weekend, that can be enough to quickly pull up an intriguing story that will blow your mind.

Don't worry! You don't have to suddenly decide that you want to be the world's greatest scientist, drop everything and create a lab in your basement advertising '*Fresh brains wanted*'. But you can tap into a whole world of free resources available to you at any given moment to help you uncover more about a topic that you find particularly interesting.

For starters, there are a lot of fascinating popular science books – like this one – out there for you to discover. Staff in any good bookstore will be delighted to be helping you discover books about your new passion, and don't get me started on libraries. Free resources and always-eager staff to help you find the current trending books. How great is that? My website has a page dedicated to giving recommendations on some of the new up-and-coming books in the field and some of the more established books in areas like neuroscience, self-help and positivity, and women in STEM. Of course, any bookstore will be able to help, but the bestsellers on Amazon will usually live up to the hype and help you to select a popular book with lots of reviews from people like yourself.

If you don't want to purchase more books, then you could try listening to podcasts in your spare time. They are becoming increasingly popular because of their varied topics and ease of use. I find them useful because I can listen to them on the move, either while commuting, walking to a store or exercising. The best thing is that with millions of podcasts to choose from, you can find one that suits your interests and your scientific background. You can literally find anything you want, which is great if you enjoy a particular area of science that doesn't have an entire book dedicated to it. Believe me, there are some seriously strange and funky podcasts out there, so give it a go – you won't be disappointed. In general, they range from basic conversations about interesting things the brain does all the way to serious and professional interviews with leading scientists.

In addition to those, and it may sound like an unlikely suggestion, but YouTube videos are a goldmine for knowledge. Sure, some videos are the scientific equivalent of voodoo and witchcraft while on psychedelic drugs, but many creators produce exceptional videos with simplified explanations that are helpful to everyone, regardless of your level of expertise. Some allow you to visualise what is happening in the human body with modern simulations and videos of how the brain works, how drugs work or how a virus tries to kill you. The simulation videos offer a viewpoint that we could never achieve in reality. Try searching for *'the inner life of the cell'* and prepare to be amazed.

There are also websites created with the sole purpose of explaining current research in a simple way that are popping up all over the place these days. It's great! They find some of the most intriguing studies that have been published recently and guide the reader through them step by step. They are a great resource if you have some free time and don't feel like taking the plunge into some of the complexities of a scientific article. Instead, they choose to dip in a toe to feel the fresh flow of science, one inch at a time. Try *'neurosciencenews.com'* to get you started.

Free online courses are, in my opinion, one of the best ways to pursue any academic interest that you have. There are literally thousands of courses to choose from, which means that you can always find a topic that is perfect for you. Formal education, such as courses taught in college and university, give structured and very inflexible programmes that inevitably have components to them that you enjoy less than others, or that you won't find useful or relevant to your personal career choice.

This is where online courses are particularly strong. They can, of course, be generalised introductions aiming to give an overall idea of the topic so you can decide whether you will find it interesting and beneficial. But they can also be very specific, enabling you to find anything from coding to cooking. This is great when you have heard about something and want to know a little more about it, or you want to become more involved in a topic that your child is learning about, helping to encourage them as you share your experiences.

Online courses are also beneficial for people who don't have a standard 9–5 schedule or are limited by work or family commitments. Free courses range from a number of weeks to many months and are fully accredited and recognised by employers. According to one poll on the *Coursera* website, a great provider of online learning, 87% of people who learn from an online course for professional development see a benefit like a raise or promotion in their current job.

Although there are thousands of free courses, those resulting in degrees will cost some money. Depending on the course, it could be in the thousands, but they are much cheaper than traditional university courses, and so still offer unbeatable value. They are a cheaper alternative not because of the quality, but because they are subsidised by private backers, charities and advertisements, in order to keep costs low.

So where do you find these courses? *Khan Academy* is a leading provider offering a wide range of courses to both kids and adults, from computer programming to science, and they even offer courses in important life skills that often go overlooked, like managing personal finances.

Coursera is another very popular choice, offering over 5,000 courses. They collaborate with more than 200 universities and employers, including Stanford University, Imperial College London and Google, and all their courses are exceptional for their level of content.

If you can't decide on the provider, *Call Central* is website that acts in a similar way to a search engine, but is specific for online courses. It directs you to any area of interest that you choose and includes courses from Harvard and MIT, which are some of the best teaching facilities in the world. What's great is that they also provide user reviews to help guide your choice. Some of the most helpful courses for a scientific career that I found were academic and essay writing courses, but there are over 30,000 on their website to choose from. Something for everybody.

If you need a starting point to find any of these platforms that work for you, I have produced lists and recommendations for everything that I have mentioned and put them on my website, which you can find details about at the back of the book.

ADVICE FOR EARLY-STAGE SCIENTISTS

In the next section, I want to share with you some tips and secrets about how you can take the next step into more advanced science. This could potentially be useful for students or anyone who wants to start a career in science, or just about anyone who wants to learn more about a topic they enjoy. It can be daunting to think of all the years of study that it takes to become an expert in your chosen field, but it doesn't have to feel that way! Together, we will take a look at some things that I'm sure every scientist wishes they had known before starting.

The most important thing, and this applies to everyone reading this, is to **find out what it is that excites you**. This sounds easier than it really is because science, even neuroscience, has many different areas to it. The best thing you can do is read around various topics, watch documentaries, reach out to people, listen to podcasts or find a research paper or two, to build an idea of what it is that you enjoy reading and learning about. Only by exposing yourself to as many different possibilities as you will you stumble upon what brings you the most joy. Often, this doesn't happen right away, and can take years to find, but only by trying out different ideas will you discover it. Maybe that is psychology (how the mind works), or researching diseases (cancer, neurodegeneration, rare diseases) or biomedical technology (you could literally build the devices of the future). Whatever it is that you enjoy doing, even if it is just a hobby, it is something that you should try to pursue.

This is not necessarily one linear process either. You may find an area that you are interested in learning about, and subsequently change your mind about it. That is perfectly fine. You only need to start looking. One thing is for certain – you don't need to decide your entire future, you only need to find your passion! Then, let it take you down the rabbit hole.

If you are studying science, at any level and at any age, then start to ask questions. Speak to course instructors, email others in the field and take advice from people working where you want to be. These are people who can give you a clearer picture of the reality of those career paths and where your potential may take you. This also helps when you are trying to build up a network of people (this will become vital within science) within a wide variety of roles who may be able to offer you indispensable insight and connections.

Another tip is that it is always worth having a look into what research is currently underway. What are the exciting new trends that are coming through? Has someone cured cancer? Do we finally have hoverboards controlled only by our thoughts? Believe me, I check for that one at least twice a week!

One great way to learn more about scientific discoveries in an area you enjoy is setting up Google alerts for trends and 'hot off the press' news. You can do this for one topic, like sleep or dreams, or you can go big and broad, and be alerted to 'neuroscience' or 'brain research'. Individual journals, where the articles are published, can also be set as alerts to focus on the field of study you are interested in. Actually, this works for anything you are curious about – it doesn't have to be about science!

Lastly, if you want to become a scientist, or if you want to work in an area you are passionate about, then getting experience in that area will really help. This may seem both obvious and impossible at the same time, as gaining initial experience is a hurdle in itself. It will not only make you more valuable as a scientist, but it will give you opportunities to try different things out, to see what you enjoy and what you definitely don't.

Summer internships or short laboratory workshops are fantastic ways to build up experience. They are designed for early-stage scientists who don't have much experience and are looking for ways to get more. Students at school or university can apply and the experiences are fantastic. I have done a few myself, and they gave me the chance to visit laboratories all over Europe.

The *Royal Society of Biology* is a UK-based charity that is involved in education, research and professional development in biology. Their summer placement programmes offer scientists an opportunity to work in all types of laboratories, both within the pharmaceutical industry and leading research groups, and offer a great route to gaining experience and confidence in science.

Biograd, a Liverpool-based institute in the UK, has courses for all levels of students and aims to have small groups with a larger number of instructors to give you a more personal and effective experience. A quick Google search will pull up these organisations and many more, and if you are not based in the UK then fear not, as other countries will their own versions. If you are in the USA, *Zippia.com* is a great tool to help search for internships; this is a search-engine type of website that enables you look for opportunities based on category and location, so you can narrow down the options to what suits you.

A more casual approach to gaining experience would be to attend networking events like *Pint of Science*, which is a worldwide science festival bringing together researchers to share their discoveries, and an amazing opportunity to speak to people in a less formal environment. Anyone can attend – you don't need to be an expert to take part. Events like these are important because, to gain experience in science, it is – and I can't stress this enough – all about networking and putting your name out there. If nothing else, it improves your conversational skills with other scientists, and at the very least, improves your confidence with small-talk, which comes in handy more often than you might think.

One thing I have seen throughout my career is the huge amount of opportunities available in research labs for people at all levels of experience. They range from full-time positions to internships or week-long work experience schemes. The initial contact is the most challenging part and will probably be more daunting than it needs to be. Emailing lecturers in universities has yielded great results for the more outgoing amongst us.

A little story about how I started. I found my way into research by reaching out and talking to a teacher in my university (where I was studying for a master's degree). We met a week later and I explained that I wanted to convert my know-how from textbooks into real research. I wanted to work in a research laboratory. The only problem was that at the time, I had no idea what that really looked like. I had worked in a hospital laboratory before, where patients' samples come through in their thousands and you help analyse them. But research? I mean, *what* was it, *where* was it, and who were these mysterious researchers working in the shadows?

I look back at this now as a rather humbling experience – it wasn't until about a year later that I realised we had the conversation *inside* a research laboratory as the teacher was actually *doing* research (he was slicing up frozen bits of spinal cord). I had no idea. He could have slapped me in the face with a lab coat and I wouldn't have noticed!

It was well worth it though, because as I explained to him how I wanted to contribute to science in the future, he listened, and then gave me the contact details of someone who he thought could really help me – another teacher at the university who had had a similar career trajectory to the one that I wanted for myself.

I got in touch, and to cut a long story short, I did a research project with that second teacher, eventually gaining a PhD in his laboratory and sealing my fate as a nerdy scientist. My dream! The point of this story is that you don't lose anything by reaching out and contacting people who might be able to give you some direction. Even if they can't assist you themselves, they might know someone else who will. This is why networking is so very important in science. At the end of the day, scientists don't get to talk about their work with as many people as you might think (usually only with other scientists anyway), so by asking questions and showing an interest you have already made their day and grown your professional network.

WHAT ELSE CAN A SCIENTIST DO?

The traditional path of a scientist is to follow the academia (university) and research route. This typically means studying up to a PhD level and conducting research in a university laboratory for several years before becoming a lecturer, then eventually a professor. Numbers of tenure-track openings have been steadily dwindling for many years, however, with less job security even for those who manage to get a position. Early-career scientists are starting to notice and look for other ways to work in science. Academia can be a great way of pursuing a scientific career, but with so many pitfalls, it is not for everyone.

Around half of all scientists in academia stay for only five years, typically the length of a laboratory position before moving into university teaching. With many scientists venturing out of the natural habitat of the lab, I felt that it is worth writing about some of the possibilities that are out there, including many that we might not expect.

186

Recent graduates from science degrees may need to broaden their search and be open to considering all positions, training and experiences in order to decide what is finally right for them. At this stage, particularly if you are a student, it is normal to feel vague about precisely how you wish to contribute to a scientific field, but it is a great time to start moving towards roles that you enjoy, with the possibility of specialising later on down the line.

It has been estimated by the US Bureau of Labor Statistics that jobs in STEM will increase by 13% over the next 10 years. The highest growth is expected to be within IT-based specialities such as software development roles, with expected growth of nearly 30%. So, what are the options if you choose to go down a non-traditional route away from the lab coat and bench?

I have spent time searching for some of the most unique and exciting roles that someone can fulfil with a background in science. Whether you opt for a graduate training programme straight out of university, or you are a postdoctoral researcher with a PhD who has decided they have had enough of lab work and want to try their hand at something a little different, the most important element that connects all of the positions is the transferable skills across even the most unusual career paths. In other words, are you someone who is good at absorbing knowledge quickly, or speaking to large crowds of people at any given moment? Perhaps you enjoy working in large interdisciplinary teams and collaborating together in an effort to produce something bigger than could be achieved alone?

Everyone has valuable skills that are unique to them, scientists and non-scientists alike. It is all about finding what makes you great and coupling that with a little creativity to find something that brings you joy. The online courses mentioned earlier are a great way to enhance your appeal by learning additional skills with a view to strengthening your interdisciplinary skill set.

So, where are all of the scientists when they are not in the laboratory?

COMMUNICATION

With a lot of science to get through, someone needs to explain it all. A science communicator is someone who does just that. This can take many forms and styles depending on what you are good at and how you like to work. Put it this way: are you bored of working in a small group and explaining your exciting and earth-shattering research only to your boss? Scientists don't have to be socially awkward human encyclopaedias, you know? They can act as the bridge between scientists and non-scientists to explain what is going on.

The more traditional way to do this would be through teaching. Either at a university, high school or some form of community college. Education careers within STEM subjects are predicted to grow by 15%, creating a strong sector that needs more educators. The US government recently invested an eye-watering $540 million into STEM education, including training and recruiting teachers.[1] Although university teaching would require PhD-level experience, schools and community colleges require a bachelor's or master's degree only. There are also options to be a specialised tutor in your preferred area of expertise, helping students to begin their own journey in science.

Science communication can mean much more than teaching, however. Perhaps becoming a science writer could open up a new way of communicating ideas from the comfort of your own computer. Writing positions vary dramatically and typically include anything from full-time writers and journalists to freelance writers for websites and magazines. The possibilities are wide-ranging, but some of the more prominent full-time writing positions can be very competitive. The growth, and therefore new posts available, is slow, and this sector is expected to shrink by 2% over the next 10 years. The good news is that further training or studying is not required in many cases, but the more writing experience you have, the better.

Scientific writing doesn't need to fall into the traditional route either. Think about biotechnology companies who need to explain what they are doing to the general public and future investors, or health services who need to communicate with the general public about their public health and outreach initiatives. If you are in interested in pharmaceuticals, there are many medical communications (*medcomms*) agencies seeking writers with in-depth knowledge of different diseases and treatment strategies. Any number of charities and organisations set up in the scientific and medical field will always need a way to talk to their audience, meaning there are opportunities to develop yourself as a science communicator here.

The Open Notebook is a scientific journalism non-profit organisation that shares tools and resources to help people to become more proficient writers about STEM subjects, and it is a great place to gain confidence and improve your skills before diving into a career change head-on.

Perhaps not what first springs to mind when discussing science communication, but science museum roles, ranging from producing displays and exhibitions to overseeing collections, has also made my list. Again, the types of available opportunities are varied but include everything from archivists to museum technicians, and may be ideal for anyone who enjoys using precise research and communication skills to express big ideas on a grand scale for larger crowds, or coming up with creative methods of storing and preserving valuable data.

Typically, a person will need a bachelor's or master's degree, and it is recommended that you gain any experience you can through training programmes or volunteering. It could be well worth doing though. The US Bureau of Labor Statistics predicts that this industry, requiring an ever-growing number of specialists, will accelerate by 11%, much faster than average, and so if it is something that you think you might enjoy, now is the time to try it out.

Business

So how about those of you who would like to hang up the lab coat to make room for a shiny suit and slicked back hair? Like it or not, science is big business. Despite the purest intentions to advance humanity and cure diseases, the reality is that there is a lot of money to be made, and the thrill of high-pressure decisions that help to make it. If you need convincing that science and business work well together, then take the example of Gordon Moore, founder of Intel, and worth an estimated $12 billion. He studied for a PhD in chemistry and went on to become successful in business and engineering.

A different type of career, far away from the lab bench, could see you using your comprehension of scientific progress for analysing business trends, particularly with pharmaceutical and biotechnology companies or consulting firms. Business analyst roles typically involve liaising with many different teams and collaborating to make the best use of market data. Scientists are valued in this industry because they can quickly assess new data and interpret their meaning. You probably already have experience in critical analysis of datasets, either for research that you have read or your own data. It is a skill that is often overlooked and sometimes undervalued, but it can be put to good use outside of the lab.

I once met someone who used their understanding of science to evaluate potential new drugs coming to market. His company would invest millions based on his feedback and assessment. It was a stressful role, but he enjoyed staying close to science while making important decisions for his company. Further training in economics and business would give you an added benefit in these types of positions, but for many, they may not be necessary.

Another side of business is sales. I mean, someone needs to tell people about new advanced equipment and drugs, right? Sales are suited more for social people who like to travel and meet new faces (maybe not ideal for those who suffer from face blindness). What is interesting about these types of positions is that sales of this nature don't use a typical door-to-door sales tactic. They generally travel to grand conferences, university labs and biotech companies, gaining exposure for new products, equipment, pharmaceuticals and medical devices.

Like with any career, if you choose a company you believe in and share their values (this may be a touchy area for pharmaceutical sales, I admit), you can sincerely be helping other institutions in their scientific efforts. Sales experience is usually required for these types of roles, but there are amazing opportunities if you can find them. It may well be worth it as the flexible working hours, autonomy and scheduling, to fit with a great work-life balance, are all qualities that have been rated highly in this type of role.[2]

ADMINISTRATION

Science isn't all lab coats and crazy hair – someone at the top needs to decide which research gets the funding to make the next big breakthrough.

Most research is funded through grants from charities, research bodies, government agencies or independent investors, and there are teams of people to help them decide where the money goes. And it is a *lot* of money. For example, the UK will be increasing its spending on research and development in STEM by 15% over the next five years, and in 2019, the total funding from the US government topped a staggering $151 billion – a steady increase of 6% from the previous year.[3]

Dealing with the decision-making power over huge sums of money will appeal to those who deal with stressful decisions especially well, but it can take a while to find a top-level position in funding agencies. They often have an extensive background in science already and use that to assess the quality and future impact of the work. Because they make recommendations on who gets the funding, scientists in this position are able to have a meaningful impact in helping to develop science and steering the future direction of research. Nevertheless, there are opportunities for graduates who would like to go down this route.

If funding puts money into basic research, then clinical trials will show you where it can end up. The typical cost of creating a new drug that successfully goes through clinical studies to reach a patient is approximately $1 billion.[4] Therefore, it is imperative that the clinical trials are done in a way that provides strong evidence that a treatment works and is safe. This requires teams of people to coordinate and log the mountains upon mountains of data and paperwork required for the regulatory approval phase, and could be an ideal option for people who have an interest in working with data like this. Working in clinical trials exposes scientists to a different aspect of research and shows the end result of what all the lonely hours in the lab can eventually lead to, i.e. helping someone get the medical treatment they need.

Why not go a step above all of these options into a role within science policy and legislature? Helping to create the rules that govern how science is conducted or deciding on strategic initiatives to improve the quality of the research will make a real difference on a national scale. These roles provide an overview of the bigger picture and allow you to see how all of the cogs work together to create a society that advances science and medicine.

Many policy positions offer graduate student programmes to attract the brightest and most talented early-career scientists. The development that is laid out by government and health agencies sets the rules for entire countries to follow. Roles here need a person who is able to communicate ideas to non-scientists in a fast-paced environment, and you could be expected to brush up on new and different topics at the drop of a hat. This may be ideal for people who work well under pressure and enjoy less of a routine work environment; instead, they are afforded the opportunity to really show their skills.

WILD CARDS

Hopefully, the positions mentioned throughout this chapter give you some idea of how you can be involved in science irrespective of where you started, helping you to see just how science research really works outside of the lab. The next section, appropriately titled as my wild cards, are written to give an idea of how wide-reaching science really is. For those who may not want a full-time career as a scientist, it will hopefully demonstrate how being open to opportunities and thinking a little creatively can lead you down a road that gives you a chance to be passionate about what you do.

Science and law actually work really well together. Patents for drugs, experimental designs, devices and almost anything you can imagine are filed every day to ensure that whoever has created a potential breakthrough product has some form of protection and rights to it. The patent office ensures that intellectual property is protected by law. At the entry level and above, law degrees are not essential, but if you have an interest in law in addition to science, then an added law degree would really launch your career forward.

Roles here are helped by the fact that the legal industry is frequently reaching out for STEM graduates to help law firms gain a market share in new areas within science. People who enjoy problem-solving, are organised with their time and can communicate their ideas well are continuously sought after.

It isn't just filing paperwork either. Within the legal industry you will find scientists advising lawyers on the specifics of scientific negotiations and licensing, ensuring that all parties understand the value in the research and legal requirements. A common feature amongst many non-traditional science careers is a good level of communication skills. Working in scientific law is no exception: a scientist essentially translates between scientists and non-scientists during discussions concerning a wide range of brand new and pioneering ideas in the field they represent.

Another type of role that makes it into the wild card list are biomedical engineering positions. This is a notoriously fast-paced area, pushing science forward either in new frontiers in AI medicine, nano-construction, surgical interventions or consumer technology. Although many people in these careers will have degrees in engineering or physics, any scientific background that adds to the understanding of new technologies is highly desired. Some of the big industry players are companies such as *Siemens Healthcare, Johnson & Johnson* and *GE Healthcare*, but the advancements in technology and an insatiable drive for consumer products mean that the number of companies that need scientists like you is always growing.

Did you ever start your science journey thinking that one day you could be a TV or movie star? OK, so this one may be a little unrealistic for most, but I wanted to explore a possibility that could be open to those who enjoy science but want to go about it in a completely different manner to the classical researcher. One prominent example would be Ken Jeong, known for his comedic role in *The Hangover* trilogy, amongst many other things. Fully trained as a medical doctor, it wasn't until later that he found his passion for acting (although he also *acts* as a doctor in TV shows).

There are openings for scientists to join in behind the scenes, for example, as a technical writer or consultant. This is a side of the industry that is expected to grow by 8% over the next 10 years, meaning potential new investment leading to more opportunities in this field. Writing or consulting for educational shows, dramas or documentaries could provide an environment that places you out of your comfort zone to research areas that you may not be familiar with. It could suit those who enjoy science communication and entertainment, although for an early-stage career change into media, it may be worth lowering initial expectations of hard-hitting shows; however, it is a fun idea nonetheless.

It is true that many career paths mentioned in this chapter require experience or further study beyond what you are interested in pursuing, but there are many that do not. Critical thinking, a strong work ethic and a confidence in your own ability will also count for a lot. Ultimately, it is fascinating to look at just how many different parts of life that science can play a role in. The skills and character traits that help you become great at what you do are important in all of these roles. They transfer over into any new position and it is always worth remembering how valuable you are, whatever you decide to do.

If nothing else, you can always write a book about the brain and neuroscience.

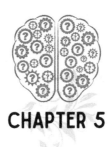

CHAPTER 5

WOMEN IN STEM

INTRODUCTION

This final chapter is something that deserves its place in this neuroscience book. It is inspired by women who continue to excel in what they do, despite any obstacles that are put before them. It is written by Jodi Barnard who has worked hard to achieve her dreams in science and will continue to impress in the future.

I wanted to include this chapter because there have been many times over the years where I have been speaking to female friends and colleagues and been surprised by their account of some of the struggles faced by being a woman working in science. From lower pay and questionable remarks, to struggling to find female role models in senior positions, there are many issues that I wish to one day understand in the hope that I can play some part in helping to improve things.

We have come a long way, but women still face stereotypes and struggles in all aspects of life, and science is no exception. I hope this section is used to spark a discussion, give some insight, or open up a new idea that you may not have read about before.

After all, science is all about asking questions. It is how we learn, improve, and continue to push the limits of what we can all do, together.

A NEUROSCIENTIST IN LONDON, WHO HAPPENS TO BE A WOMAN

By Jodi Barnard

Jodi here! I am a neuroscience PhD student in London, using human cells in a dish to study the way our neurons interact with immune cells in the brain to cause inflammation and cell death in diseases such as Alzheimer's. I am also using fruit flies to research human genes related to Motor Neuron Disease. But I haven't always been in this place. I came from a low socio-economic background, working since the age of 13. I know what it is to worry about money. This is one of the things that drove me to do well at school. This, and the stubbornness that years of bullying instils in you. When you are told you can't, you want to show you can. Despite the barriers.

As the first in my family to go to university, I had no clue what I was supposed to be doing. It seemed everyone around me had a plan and I was just fumbling along in the dark only seeing the next step when I was about to stumble over it. I liked science, but I didn't know you could be a scientist. I thought if you were interested in biology you become a medical doctor.

As a girl I also felt less encouraged to pursue science - even being told by my science teacher that I "should stick to poetry". But all these things spurred me on. On top of being working class, first-gen and female, my home life and the night shifts I was working at the hospital, made studying from home difficult. Then, during High school I was very unwell - one emergency surgery later - and I did not meet my entry requirements for medical school. My world crumbled. Without proper careers guidance I accepted the first course I was offered - this was Medical Neuroscience at Sussex. And so, I sort of fell into neuroscience and I fell in love.

But this isn't the end of the 'success story'. Things continued to be difficult. I worked throughout university just to afford to live. I suffered with my mental health and with more medical school rejections, I wasn't sure what I was supposed to be doing. So, when I was offered a scholarship toward a master's course, I took it. Working long hours in the lab on top of a part-time job, I experienced my first episode of burnout.

But I did love being in the lab and so I decided to apply for a PhD - after all I had a faultless academic record. But I was rejected from every program and my imposter syndrome hit hard. I couldn't afford to reapply; my housing tenancy came to an end and the 'uni bubble' popped. I needed an income.

I started working for a wearable technology company. Often, I was the only woman in the room, and I felt so undervalued and out of my depth. My anxiety worsened to the point where I knew I needed to get back to what made me happy. I secured a research assistant job and I loved working in the lab again. I was sure I wanted to do a PhD this time and I threw every ounce of energy into many applications and interviews, until I got my offer from King's College London, a top university.

You see, there's no wrong path into STEM. These experiences collectively make me very aware of the challenges people from under-represented groups face and is the reason why I co-host an equality in STEM podcast, The Academinist, and work with organisations which aim to improve access to higher education. All these experiences have developed a resilience in me. The ability to pick myself back up and try again has been invaluable in getting to where I am, and I am sure will continue to serve me well as I work toward my PhD. The sense of achievement I get from conquering something challenging is what I love most about what I do. That, and the ability to be creative and continue to learn, all whilst trying to better humanity. This is why I am a scientist.

The Covid-19 pandemic has exposed inequalities affecting women, such as the second shift phenomena whereby caring responsibilities (often falling to women) and unpaid labour in the home stack on top of the usual workday. Alessandra Minello wrote about the maternal wall blocking faculty advancement for women in a scientific publication around the start of the first UK lockdown in 2020.[1] Since then, analyses on several medical journals have revealed a so-called Covid-19 effect whereby the proportion of female authors is lower than the average.[2] This links to other challenges that existed before Covid-19, such as the complexities of having a career and a family. For me, this is always something in the back of my mind. Hearing the thumping tick of my biological clock - as if it is a race against time to get to a position in my career where having a family will have minimal impact on my prospects. Of course, not all women want/can have children, but for those of us whom this is a priority, it is tiring to constantly feel like you are justifying your choices to others/society/yourself. I have spoken to women who have witnessed awful comments and micro-aggressions toward pregnant women and mothers in academia. For me, another change is much more imminent - I am due to get married next year and I am even worrying about the name change and the impact it will have on the reputation I have worked so hard to build up. These are just some of extra stresses that are somewhat unique to women in STEM.

Another issue, and the idea behind the 'this is what a scientist looks like' movement, is the stereotypical view of the women who work in STEM. Interestingly, these views are not always held by men. There's a common narrative that you need to be a certain type of woman to fit into that space e.g. geeky, 'plain Jane', or basically Amy Farrah Fowler from The Big Bang Theory. And so, it is not enough to say 'women don't want to work in science' - it is about showcasing that all women belong in science. The idea of being a multi-faceted human first and a scientist second, is the way forward. Maybe then, more young girls and women would self-identify as being 'cut out' for this profession. We need to be encouraging more diversity into these fields – invaluable work is being done by charities such as *I Can Be* to increase the visibility of job opportunities to young girls. This can only solve one issue, because plenty of women do make it to the PhD level and above, but very few women can be found in higher positions. This leaky pipeline problem needs addressing because without representative role models in higher positions, it is hard for women to keep up with the workload knowing that our chances of reaching the top of that ladder are slim.

Personally, the women in STEM within the social media community and the scientists I work with, have been an invaluable female support system for me. I haven't had any formal female mentors, but I feel I could have benefitted from this, which is why I try to mentor as many young women as possible in my spare time. I feel it is necessary that we pull each other up.

But it isn't all doom and gloom. We are seeing progress around us every day. Most recently, with inspiring women like Emmanuelle Charpentier and Jennifer A. Doudna being awarded the 2020 Nobel Prize in Chemistry "for the development of a method for genome editing", creating role models for young girls and women. The only way we can fix the problems that persist is by moving forward together, all genders. With discussion, education, and awareness, the 'not our problem' attitude that sometimes makes conversations such as these seem optional, will dissolve. Initiatives which are held up by 'woman power' and the efforts of minority groups, will become a shared burden. More urgently, we need to put more weight onto initiatives which reach out to young girls and encourage entry to STEM, outreach and mentoring work. Using these activities alongside the current metrics a scientist is judged on, such as the number of publications, will allow us to assess things like fair pay and suitability for promotion more accurately.

So, although some challenges remain, the progress that continues to be made fills me with optimism for the future of women and non-binary people occupying spaces in STEM, and I for one, will continue to do all that I can to shout as loudly as I can about them.

AFTERWORD

Thank you for reading my book. I really hope that you enjoyed it and learned something new about how amazing the brain is, and how exciting neuroscience can be.

It has been an incredible experience writing this book taking you on a journey through the brain and neuroscience. If I could ask one favour? Please could you leave a review on Amazon. I rely on reviews to help people decide whether or not they should read my book and it really does help me in a very real way. I appreciate it so much, thank you.

If you have any questions about what you have read, then drop me an email or message using the website or Instagram page, I would love to hear from you. The website also contains lots of useful suggestions for how you can keep going on your neuroscience journey, so please make sure to have a look.

www.aNeuroRevolution.com
Instagram: @TheEnglishScientist

If you enjoyed the women in STEM chapter then you can follow the author on social media or listen to her podcast.

Jodi Barnard, née Parslow
Instagram & Twitter: @notbrainscience
Podcast: https://theacademinist.buzzsprout.com/

Thank you again for reading and supporting this book.

Acknowledgments

I would like to give a big thank you to my friends and family who helped me to shape the text into something even better. A special thanks to Diana Carter, who I have now labelled as my unofficial editor during those times when I was stressed that my writing was smouldering hot science trash, and to Ike dela Peña PhD, for his scientific editing of specific sections. A thank you to Kate Linge for her technical expertise.

I also want to mention Dr Matt Bolland, Thomas Gatti, Farah Ghosn, Cian McGuire PhD, and Sagar Raturi PhD, and Andy Tranter, who read through some early drafts to make sure I wasn't writing nonsense, and Steph Tranter who helped me to use social media. There is a thank you that also needs to go out to Sara Solak, AKA 'The Cookie Lady' (Instagram @cpmfcookiesandcrafts) for patiently listening to me talk about nothing else but my book for the last six months, and to Amanda Limonius for listening to my last minute writing rants. Of course, I want to thank Melissa Estrada for encouraging me throughout the entire process, helping me to make the book what it is today.

Finally, I would like to thank you, the reader, for taking the time to read my book and for going on this journey through neuroscience with me.

Glossary

Aβ PEPTIDE Amyloid beta, part of the amyloid plaques that are involved in Alzheimer's disease. A peptide is a short sequence of amino acids that make up a protein

AI Simulating human intelligence and thinking in a programmed machine, artificial intelligence

AMPA Receptors most widely known for their glutamate binding in learning and memory, alpha-amino-3-hydroxy-5-methyl-4-isoxazolepropionic acid

AMYGDALA An area in the temporal lobe which plays an integral part of the behaviour and emotional centre, the limbic system

ANTERIOR CINGULATE CORTEX (ACC) Frontal region of the cingulate cortex involved in empathy, decision-making, and executive control over many other brain functions

ASTROCYTE A subtype of glial cells, this star-shaped cell has complex functions including maintaining neuronal synapses

BCI A communication between the brain and a computerised device to enable or enhance brain function

BIOMARKER Something that is used as an indicator of a biological process. An example would be a protein that can be measured to understand a disease progression

CAUDATE NUCLEUS Near the centre of the brain, it is involved in movement, planning, memory, addiction, and emotions

CIRCADIAN RHYTHM Biological activity of the body that occurs within a 24-hour cycle

CONNECTIONS Linking of neurons with others to form a network of communication

CORTEX The outer layer of the brain, basically the visible part that you can see

CRISPR A gene editing technique, Clusters of Regularly Interspaced Short Palindromic Repeats

CRYPTOCHROME A protein sensitive to light and involved in sensing magnetic fields

DECLARATIVE MEMORY A type of long-term memory for facts and events that we are consciously aware of

DENDRITE A branch, or extension, of a neuron

DENTATE GYRUS A structure within the hippocampus involved in helping to coordinate memories

DNA The instructions for the life of a cell, that are stored in the nucleus of every cell in the body, deoxyribonucleic acid

EEG A non-invasive measure of brain waves, electroencephalogram

ELECTRODE A small device to record electrical activity

FUSIFORM GYRUS Plays a big role in recognising faces and facial expressions

GABA An inhibitory neurotransmitter, gamma aminobutyric acid

GLIAL CELLS Support cells to neurons which include astrocytes, oligodendrocytes, microglia, and ependymal cells

GYRUS Rounded folds on the surface of the brain to increase surface area for more neurons

HIPPOCAMPUS A sea-horse shaped band in the temporal lobe critical in learning and creating memories

HPA AXIS Linked regions that control stress through hormones and brain responses, hypothalamic-pituitary-adrenal

HYPOTHALAMUS Control centre for the nervous system and things like body temperature

ION CHANNEL A cell surface channel (protein) that allows the passage of ions in and out of the cell

LIMBIC SYSTEM A collection of structures including the amygdala, hippocampus, hypothalamus, tegmentum, OFC, and ACC, that influence behaviour and emotions

LOCUS COERULEUS Produces the neurotransmitter, noradrenaline, involved in many things, such as attention levels

LONG–TERM DEPRESSION A process to reduce the efficiency of neurons in order to forget, primarily for motor movements

LONG–TERM POTENTIATION A process to increase the efficiency of neurons and their connections to facilitate memories

LUCID DREAM A dream in which the person gains an awareness of the dream

MRI Imaging to see the body and brain, magnetic resonance imaging

NAV An ion channel that prefers to let sodium ions pass through

NEOCORTEX The newest part of the brain to form and involved in things like decision-making and language

NEURODEGENERATION A condition in which part of the nervous system, such as a neuron, loses its function and structure, and no longer works properly

NEURON A type of cell to transmit a signal

NEUROTRANSMITTER A chemical messenger between neurons

NOCICEPTOR Receptors than transmit pain, and the neurons that contain them are referred to as nociceptors

NMDA A stimulatory neurotransmitter, N-methyl-D-aspartate

NON-DECLARATIVE MEMORY A type of long-term memory that occurs without our conscious awareness, such as remembering how to walk or ride a bike

NREM SLEEP Non-rapid eye movement phase during sleep

NUCLEUS ACCUMBENS An area involved in dopamine signalling for movement and addiction

ORGANOID A simple version of an organ, made up of cells, and studied in the laboratory

PREOPTIC ANTERIOR HYPOTHALAMUS (POAH) An area of the hypothalamus that regulates temperature

PLASTICITY A modified brain structure to alter its function

PREFRONTAL CORTEX (PFC) Front part of the brain involved in higher, executive functions, like prediction, planning, and generally involved in many behaviours of the brain

RECEPTOR A protein structure on the surface of a cell to receive a signal and convert that to a message inside the cell

REM SLEEP Rapid eye movement during sleep

STEM CELLS The special 'new' cells that can eventually be any type of cell in the body

SUBTHALAMIC NUCLEUS (STN) A small number of neurons below the thalamus that contributes to movement but may be involved in decision-making and memory

SUBSTANTIA NIGRA (SN) A region in the midbrain that contains dopamine and melanin neurons important in Parkinson's disease and the reward pathway

SUPRACHIASMATIC NUCLEUS (SCN) Within the hypothalamus it serves as the pacemaker for the circadian rhythm

SYNAPSE The gap between neurons where neurotransmitters are released

THALAMUS A small area just above the brain stem which acts as the relay centre for messages getting into the brain

VENTRAL TEGMENTAL AREA (VTA) A midbrain structure that projects dopamine neurons, heavily involved in movement, motivation, and reward pathways

VENTROLATERAL PREOPTIC NUCLEUS (VLPO) Important in controlling sleep predominantly through a system of inhibitory neurons

References

CHAPTER 1: Ask a neuroscientist
What is the oldest part of our brain, and what does it do

1. MacLean, P. (1990). *The triune brain in evolution: Role in paleocerebral functions*. Plenum, New York.

What does cannabis actually do to my brain, should I be worried?

2. Malone, *et al.* (2010). Adolescent cannabis use and psychosis: epidemiology and neurodevelopmental model. *Br J Pharm*; 160 (3).

3. Colizzi, *et al.* (2015). Interaction between functional genetic variation of DRD2 and cannabis use on risk of psychosis. *Schiz Bull*; 41 (5).

4. Eldreth, *et al.* (2004). Abnormal brain activity in prefrontal brain regions in abstinent marijuana users. *Neuroimage*; 23 (3).

5. de Souza Crippa, *et al.* (2004). Effect of cannabidiol (CBD) on regional cerebral blood flow. *Neuropsychopharm*; 29 (2).

6. Masataka (2019). Anxiolytic effects of repeated cannabidiol treatment in teenagers with social anxiety disorders. *Front Psychol*; 10.

7. Skelley, *et al.* (2003). Use of cannabidiol in anxiety and anxiety-related disorders. *J AM Pharm Assoc*; 60 (1).

Why do we seem to 'click' with some people and become instant friends?

8. Tseng, *et al.* (2018). Interbrain cortical synchronization encodes multiple aspects of social interactions in monkey pairs. *Scientific Reports*; 8 (4699).

9. Lee, *et al.* (2015). Emergence of the default-mode network from resting-state to activation-state in reciprocal social interaction via eye contact. *Annu Int Conf IEEE Eng Med Biol Soc*; 2015.

10. di Pellegrino, *et al.* (1992). Understanding motor events: a neurophysiological study. *Exp Brain Res*; 91 (1).

11. Molenberghs, *et al.* (2012). Brain regions with mirror properties: a meta-analysis of 125 human fMRI studies. *Neurosci Biobehav Rev*; 36 (1).

12. Khalil, *et al.* (2018). Social decision making in autism: On the impact of mirror neurons, motor control, and imitative behaviors. *CNS Neurosci Ther*; 24 (8).

Does learning extra languages impact other brain functions and memory?

13. Javor (2016). Bilingualism, theory of mind and perspective-taking: the effect of early bilingual exposure. *Psychol & Behav Sci*; 5 (6).

14. Craik, *et al.* (2010). Delaying the onset of Alzheimer's disease – bilingualism as a form of cognitive reserve. *Neurology*; 75 (19).

15. Alladi, *et al.* (2016). Impact of Bilingualism on Cognitive Outcome After Stroke. *Stroke*; 47 (1).

Why do we get addicted to things?

16. Volkow, *et al.* (2011). Reward, dopamine and the control of food intake: implications for obesity. *Trends Cogn Sci*; 15 (1).

17. Schultz, (1998). Predictive reward signal of dopamine neurons. *J Neurophsy*; 80 (1).

18. Elliot, *et al.* (2003). Differential response patterns in the striatum and orbitofrontal cortex to financial reward in humans: a parametric functional magnetic resonance imaging study. *J Neurosci*; 23 (1).

19. Ducci & Goldman (2012). The genetic basis of addictive disorders. *Psych Clin North Am*; 35 (2).

Why do we get memory loss when we hit our head?

20. Vakil (2005). The effect of moderate to severe traumatic brain injury (TBI) on different aspects of memory: a selective review. *J Clin Exp Neuropsychol*; 27.

21. Rigon, *et al.* (2019). Procedural memory following moderate-severe traumatic brain injury: group performance and individual differences on the rotary pursuit task. *Front Human Neurosci*; 13 (251).

What is sleep, and why do we do it?

22. Hoevenaar-Blom, *et al.* (2011). Sleep duration and sleep quality in relation to 12-year cardiovascular disease incidence: the MORGEN study. *Sleep*; 34.

23. Musiek & Holtzman (2016). Mechanisms linking circadian clocks, sleep, and neurodegeneration. *Science*; 354 (6315).

24. Carlson & Chiu (2008). The absence of circadian cues during recovery

from sepsis modifies pituitary-adrenocortical function and impairs survival. *Shock*; 29.

25. Mainieri, *et al.* (2020). Are sleep paralysis and false awakenings different from REM sleep and from lucid REM sleep? A spectral EEG analysis. *J Clin Sleep Med*; epub 2020.

What are dreams, and why do we have them?

26. Hajek & Belcher (1991). Dream of absent-minded transgression: an empirical study of a cognitive withdrawal symptom. *J Abnorm Psychol*; 100 (4).

27. Wamsley & Stickgold (2011). Memory, sleep and dreaming: experiencing consolidation. *Sleep Med Clin*; 6 (1).

28. Stickgold, *et al.* (2000). Replaying the game: hypnagogic images in normal and amnesics. *Science*; 290.

29. Paulson, *et al.* (2017). Dreaming: a gateway to the unconscious? *Annals of the New York Academy of Sciences*; 1406.

30. Nielsen & Stentstrom (2005). What are the memory sources of dreaming? *Nature*; 437 (7063).

31. Levin & Nielsen (2007) Disturbed dreaming posttraumatic stress disorder, and affect distress: A review and neurocognitive model. *Psychol Bull*; 133 (3).

32. Baird, *et al.* (2019). The cognitive neuroscience of lucid dreaming. *Neurosci Biobehav Rev*; 100.

33. Spoormaker & van den Bout (2006). Lucid dreaming treatment for nightmares: a pilot study. *Psychotherapy & Psychosomatics*; 75 (6).

34. Baird, *et al.* (2018). Frequent lucid dreaming associated with increased functional connectivity between frontopolar cortex and temporoparietal association areas. *Scientific Reports*; 8.

35. LaBerge, *et al.* (2018) Pre-sleep treatment with galantamine stimulates lucid dreaming: a double-blind, placebo-controlled, crossover study. *PLoS ONE*; 13.

36. Konkoly, *et al.* (2021). Real-time dialogue between experimenters and dreamers during REM sleep. *Current Biology*; 31.

Can brain cells regenerate?

37. Moreno-Jiménez, *et al.* (2019). Adult hippocampal neurogenesis is abundant in neurologically healthy subjects and drops sharply in patients with Alzheimer's disease. *Nature Medicine*; 25.

38. Gunnar, *et al.* (2020). Injured adult neurons regress to an embryonic transcriptional growth state. *Nature*; 581 (7806).

39. Reimer, *et al.* (2008). Motor Neuron Regeneration in Adult Zebrafish. *J Neuroscience*; 28 (34).

How are memories encoded in the brain?

40. Wixted, *et al.* (2014). Sparse and distributed coding of episodic memory in neurons of the human hippocampus. *PNAS*; 111 (26).

41. Müller, *et al.* (2017). Hippocampal-caudate nucleus interactions support exceptional memory performance. *Brain Struct Funct*; 223.

Does a genius have a different brain?

42. Goriounova, *et al.* (2018). Large and fast human pyramidal neurons associate with intelligence. *Elife*; 7.

43. Pietschnig, *et al.* (2015). Meta-analysis of association between human brain volume and intelligence differences: How strong are they and what do they mean? *Neuroscience and Behavioural Reviews*; 57.

44. Hilger, *et al.* (2017). Intelligence is associated with the modular structure of intrinsic brain networks. *Scientific Reports*; 7.

45. Catani & Mazzarello. (2019). Leonardo da Vinci: a genius driven to distraction. *Brain*; 142 (6).

Can the brain really multitask?

46. Madore & Wagner (2019). Multicosts of multitasking. *Cerebrum*; 1.

47. Clapp, *et al.* (2011). Deficit in switching between functional brain networks underlies the impact of multitasking on working memory in older adults. *PNAS*; 108 (9170).

What is depression, and does it change the brain?

48. Hasin, *et al.* (2018). Epidemiology of adult DSM-5 major depressive disorder and Its specifiers in the United States. *JAMA Psychiatry*; 75 (4).

49. Davis, *et al.* (2020). Effects of psilocybin-assisted therapy on major depressive disorder. *JAMA Psychiatry*; epub 2020.

50. Stockmeier, *et al.* (2004). Cellular changes in the postmortem hippocampus in major depression. *Biol Psychiatry*; 56 (9).

51. Ménard, *et al.* (2016). Pathogenesis of depression: insights from human and rodent studies. *Neuroscience*; 321.

52. Fang, *et al.* (2020). Chronic unpredictable stress induces depression-

related behaviors by suppressing AgRP neuron activity. *Mol Psychiatry*; 1.

53. Lutz, et al. (2017). Association of a history of child abuse with impaired myelination in the anterior cingulate cortex: convergent epigenetic, transcriptional, and morphological evidence. Am J Psychiatry; 174 (12).

54. Sarris, *et al.* (2014). Lifestyle medication for depression. *BMC Psychiatry*; 14 (107).

55. Gujral, *et al.* (2017). Exercise effects on depression: possible neural mechanisms. *Gen Hosp Psychiatry*; 49.

56. Nokia, *et al.* (2016). Physical exercise increases adult hippocampal neurogenesis in male rats provided it is aerobic and sustained. *J Phys*; 594 (7).

57. Ambrosi, *et al.* (2019). Randomized controlled study on the effectiveness of animal-assisted therapy on depression, anxiety, and illness perception in institutionalized elderly. *Psychogeriatrics*; 19 (1).

What happens in the brain during meditation, are there any real benefits?

58. Vasudev, *et al.* (2016). A training programme involving automatic self-transcending meditation in late-life depression: preliminary analysis of an ongoing randomised controlled trial. *B J Psych Open*; 2 (2).

59. Kuyken, *et al.* (2015). Effectiveness and cost-effectiveness of mindfulness-based cognitive therapy compared with maintenance antidepressant treatment in the prevention of depressive relapse or recurrence (PREVENT): a randomised controlled trial. *Lancet*; 386 (9988).

60. Goyal, *et al.* (2014). Meditation programs for psychological stress and well-being: a systematic review and meta-analysis. *JAMA Intern Med;* 174 (3).

61. Wielgosz, *et al.* (2019). Mindfulness meditation and psychopathology. *Ann Rev Clin Psychol*; 15.

62. Schlosser, *et al.* (2019). Unpleasant meditation-related experiences in regular meditators: prevalence, predictors, and conceptual considerations. *PLOS One*; 14 (5).

Do men and women have different brains?

63. Ingalhalikar, *et al.* (2014). Sex differences in the structural connectome of the human brain. *PNAS*; 111 (2).

64. Zhang, *et al.* (2020). Gender differences are encoded differently in the structure and function of human brain revealed by multimodal MRI. *Front Human Neuro*; 14 (244).

65. Caplan, *et al.* (2017). Do microglia play a role in sex differences in TBI? *J Neuro Research*; 95.

66. Lotze, *et al.* (2019). Novel findings from 2,838 adult brains on sex differences in gray matter brain volume. *Scientific Reports*; 9 (1671).

67. Liutsko, *et al.* (2020). Fine motor precision tasks: sex differences in performance with and without visual guidance across different age groups. *Behav Sci*; 10 (1).

68. Nieuwenhuis, *et al.* (2017). Multi-center MRI prediction models: predicting sex and illness course in first episode psychosis patients. *Neuroimage*; 145 (pt2).

69. Sommer, *et al.* (2008). Sex differences in handedness, asymmetry on the planum temporale and functional language lateralization. *Brain Research*; 1206.

70. McDaniel (2005). Big-brained people are smarter: a meta-analysis of the relationship between in vivo brain volume and intelligence. *Intelligence*; 33 (4).

71. Pietschnig, *et al.* (2015). Meta-analysis of associations between human brain volume and intelligence differences: How strong are they and what do they mean? *Neurosci & Behav Rev*; 57.

What is our consciousness?

72. Hudetz, *et al.* (2015). Dynamic repertoire of intrinsic brain states is reduced in propofol-induced unconsciousness. *Brain Connect*; 5 (1).

73. Libet, *et al.* (1983). Time of conscious intention to act in relation to onset of cerebral activity (readiness-potential). The unconscious initiation of a freely voluntary act. *Brain*; 106 (pt 3).

74. Matsuhashi & Hallet. (2008). The timing of conscious intention to move. *Eur J Neuro*; 28 (11).

CHAPTER 2: The X-Files of neuroscience

1. Enoch & Trethowan (1991). *Uncommon psychiatric syndromes*. (3rd ed), Oxford, Boston; Butterworht-Heinemann.

2. Hirstein & Ramachandran (1997). Capgras syndrome: a novel probe for understanding the neural representation of the identity and familiarity of persons. *Proc Biol Sci*; 264 (1380).

3. Caputo (2010). Strange-face-in-the-mirror-illusion. *Perception*; 39.

4. Caputo (2015). Dissociation and hallucinations in dyads engaged through interpersonal gazing. *Psychiatry Research*; 228.

5. Grossi, *et al.* (2014). Structural connectivity in a single case of progressive prosopagnosia: the role of the right inferior longitudinal fasciculus. *Cortex*; 56.

6. Petrone, *et al.* (2020). Preservation of neurons in an AD 79 vitrified human brain. *PLoS ONE*; 15 (10).

7. Hames, *et al.* (2012). An urge to jump affirms the urge to live: an empirical examination of the high places phenomenon. *Journal of Affective Disorders*; 136.

8. Wang, *et al.* (2019). Transduction of the geomagnetic field as evidence from alpha-band activity in the human brain. *eNeuro*; 6 (2).

9. Weiskrantz, *et al.* (1974). Visual capacity in the hemianopic field following a restricted occipital ablation. *Brain*; 97 (4).

10. Ajina, *et al.* (2020). The superior colliculus and amygdala support evaluation of face trait in blindsight. *Front Neurol*; 11 (769).

11. Linda Rodriguez McRobbie (2017). Total recall: the people who never forget. The Guardian Newspaper; 8 February. https://www.theguardian.com/science/2017/feb/08/total-recall-the-people-who-never-forget.

12. Santangelo, *et al.* (2018). Enhanced brain activity associated with memory access in highly superior autobiographical memory. *PNAS*; 115 (30).

CHAPTER 3: The future of neuroscience

1. Ian Sample (2012). The Guardian Newspaper. Harvard University says it can't afford journal publishers' prices. 24 April. https://www.theguardian.com/science/2012/apr/24/harvard-university-journal-publishers-prices.

2. Anna Fazackerley (2021). The Guardian Newspaper. Price gouging from Covid: student ebooks costing up to 500% more than in print. 29 January. https://www.theguardian.com/education/2021/jan/29/price-gouging-from-covid-student-ebooks-costing-up-to-500-more-than-in-print.

3. de Vries, *et al* (2019). A large-scale standardized physiological survey reveals functional organization of the mouse visual cortex. *Nature Neuroscience*; 23.

4. Wu, *et al.* (2020). Kilohertz two-photon fluorescence microscopy imaging of neural activity in vivo. *Nature Methods*; 17 (3).

5. Weisenburger, *et al.* (2019). Volumetric Ca2+ imaging in the mouse brain using hybrid multiplexed sculpted light microscopy. *Cell*; 177 (4).

6. Gao, *et al.* (2019). Cortical column and whole-brain imaging with molecular contrast and nanoscale resolution. *Science*; 363 (6424).

7. Antonio Regalado (2018). https://www.technologyreview.com/2018/03/13/144721/a-startup-is-pitching-a-mind-uploading-service-that-is-100-percent-fatal/.

8. White, *et al* (1971). Primate cephalic transplantation: neurogenic separation, vascular association. *Transpl Proc*; 3.

9. Oxley, *et al.* (2020). Motor neuroprosthesis implanted with neurointerventional surgery improves capacity for activities of daily living tasks in severe paralysis: first in-human experience. *J Neurointervent Surg*.

10. Kangassalo, *et al.* (2020). Neuroadaptive modelling for generating images matching perceptual categories. *Scientific Reports*; 10.

11. Jiang, *et al.* (2019). BrainNet: A multi-person brain-to-brain interface for direct collaboration between brains. *Scientific Reports*; 9 (6115).

12. Chiaradia & Lancaster (2020). Brain organoids for the study of human neurobiology at the interface of in vitro and in vivo. *Nature Neuroscience*; 23.

13. Kim, *et al.* (2015). A 3D human neural cell culture system for modelling Alzheimer's disease. *Nat Protoc*; 10 (7).

14. Cairns, *et al* (2020). A 3D human brain-like tissue model of herpes-induced Alzheimer's disease. *Science Advances*; 6.

15. Todhunter, *et al.* (2015). Programmed synthesis of three-dimensional tissues. *Nature Methods*; 12 (10).

16. Food and Drug Administration November 6, 2020: https://www.fda.gov/advisory- committees/advisory-committee-calendar/november-6-2020-meeting-peripheral-and-central-nervous-system-drugs-advisory-committee-meeting.

17. Jinek, *et al.* (2012). A programmable dual-RNA–guided DNA endonuclease in adaptive bacterial immunity. *Science*; 337.

18. Barrangou, *et al.* (2016). Applications of CRISPR technologies in research and beyond. *Nat Biotechnol*; 34.

19. Sanders, *et al* (2014). LRRK2 mutations cause mitochondrial DNA damage in iPSC-derived neural cells from Parkinson's disease patients: reversal by gene correction. *Neurobiol Dis*; 62.

20. Jonsson, *et al.* (2012). A Mutation in APP protects against Alzheimer's disease and age-related cognitive decline. *Nature*; 488.

21. Firth, *et al.* (2015). Functional gene correction for cystic fibrosis in lung epithelial cells generated from patient iPSCs. *Cell Rep*; 12 (9).

22. Osborn, *et al.* Fanconi anemia gene editing by the CRISPR/Cas9 system.

Human Gene Therapy; 26.

23. Fan, *et al.* (2018). The role of gene editing in neurodegenerative disease. *Cell Transplant*; 27 (3).

24. Sermer & Brentjens (2019). CAR T-cell therapy: full speed ahead. *Hematol Oncol*; 37 (supp 1).

25. Ma, *et al.* (2017). Corrections of a pathogenic gene mutation in human embryos. *Nature*; 548.

26. Ewen Callaway (2018). Did CRISPR really fix a genetic mutation in these human embryos? 08 Aug. Nature: https://www.nature.com/articles/d41586-018-05915-2.

27. Allen, *et al.* (2018). Predicting the mutations generated by repair of Cas9-induced double-strand breaks. *Nature Biotechnology*; 37.

28. Campa, *et al* (2019). Multiplexed genome engineering by Cas12a and CRISPR arrays encoded on single transcripts. *Nature Methods*; 16.

29. Basil Leaf Technologies. December 21 2020. www.basilleaftech.com/dxter.

30. Pais-Vieira, *et al.* (2013). A Brain-to-brain interface for real-time sharing of sensorimotor information. *Scientific Reports*; 3 (1319).

31. Onestack, (1997). The effect of visual-motor behavior rehearsal (VMBR) and videotaped modelling on the free-throw performance of intercollegiate athletes. *Journal of Sport Behavior*; 1.

32. Ranganathan, *et al.* (2004). From mental power to muscle power – gaining strength by using the mind. *Neuropsychologia*; 42.

33. Hampson, *et al.* (2018). Developing a hippocampal neural prosthetic to facilitate human memory encoding and recall. *J Neural Eng*; 15 (3).

CHAPTER 4: Down the science rabbit-hole

1. U.S. Department of Education. Nov 2019. https://www.ed.gov/news/press-releases/us-department-education-advances-trump-administrations-stem-investment-priorities.

2. Med Reps. 2019. 2019 9th annual medical sales salary report. https://www.medreps.com/medical-sales-careers/2019-medical-sales-salary-report.

3. Office for national statistics. (2020). Research and development expenditure by the UK government. https://www.ons.gov.uk/economy/governmentpublicsectorandtaxes/research

anddevelopmentexpenditure/bulletins/ukgovernmentexpenditureonsciencee
ngineeringandtechnology/2018.

4. Wouters, *et al.* (2020). Estimated research and development investment
needed to bring a new medicine to market, 2009-2018. *JAMA*; 323 (9).

CHAPTER 5: Women in STEM

A neuroscientist in London, who happens to be a woman by Jodi Barnard

1. Minello. (2020). The pandemic and the female academic. *Nature*;
17.

2. Viglione. (2020). Are women publishing less during the pandemic? Here's
what the data say. *Nature*; 581 (7809).

EXTRAS

Image attribution for Phineas Gage

Originally from the collection of Jack and Beverly Wilgus, and now in the
Warren Anatomical Museum, Harvard Medical School.

Hello there.

You made it all the way to the back of the book, and even through the reference pages!

That's great. Thank you for reading it all.

But now there is no more.

Or is there..........

Nope, it's all gone.

Made in United States
North Haven, CT
27 December 2022

30243730R00127